ANTICANCER BOTANICALS

ANTICANCER BOTANICALS

by

Sukanya Bhattacharya

Head, Department of Botany,

Vidyasagar College, Kolkata

2006

DAYA PUBLISHING HOUSE

DELHI-110 035

ISBN 81-7035-383-1

Published by : **Daya Publishing House**
1123/74, Deva Ram Park
Tri Nagar, Delhi-110 035
Phone : 27103999
Fax : (011) 27199029
E-mail : dayabooks@vsnl.com
Website : www.dayabooks.com

Showroom : 4760-61/23, Ansari Road
New Delhi - 110 002
Ph.: 23245578, 23244987

Laser Composed by : **Vaishnav Graphics & Systems**
New Delhi - 110 055

Printed at : **Chawla Offset Printers**
Delhi-110 052

PRINTED IN INDIA

Dedicated to the memory of my beloved
Dida and Dadu

A light from our midst is gone,
A voice we loved is stilled,
A place is vacant in our home,
Which never can be filled.

Dadu,

You fell asleep without a good bye,
The memories we share will never die.

Preface

During the last decade, chemical carcinogenesis research has made substantial progress and has provided the impetus for a cure of the dreaded disease. The story of the development of anticancer drugs is one of steady progress rather than sudden dramatic development.

Central to the problem of curing, is an understanding of the ways in which normal and cancer cells differ. The book has provided adequate information concerning the biochemical and regression characteristics of pre-neoplasia in a precisely defined model of experimental hepatocarcinogenesis.

The book explains and emphasizes the effective role of the plant extracts in maintaining the antioxidant defence and hepatic biotransformation system and discusses the impact of its contribution to the suppression of aberrant function of cells associated with the killer disease. The survival of the animals in presence and absence of plant extracts has been correlated with the biochemical basis of neoplasticity. Histopathological and ultrastructural techniques have been used to confirm the chemopreventive efficacy of the plant extract.

The accumulating knowledge of cellular processes from this work can be beneficial to the ultimate aim of achieving a cure for Hepatic cancer particularly in view of its rapid incidence in this part of the world.

Acknowledgements

I would like to take this privilege of offering my sincere gratitude to the Council of Scientific and Industrial Research (C.S.I.R.), Government of India for providing me the necessary grant to carry out the Research project during my tenure as J.R.F. (NET) and S.R.F. (NET). I am highly indebted to Prof S. Som, V.C., Mr. R. Banerjee, Registrar of Jadavpur University for extending to me all necessary facilities during the entire course of experimentation.

I am specially thankful to Prof. Dr. Subir Dutta, Dean, Faculty of Medicine, Calcutta University, Dr. A.N. Basu, Dean Faculty of Science, J.U, Dr. S.B. Mahato, Emeritus Scientist, C.S.I.R., I.I.C.B., Calcutta. I express my heartfelt gratitude to Dr. Subir Dutta for his excellent suggestions and critical interpretation of histochemical results related to the present work.

It is my great pleasure to mention the untiring help and valuable suggestions of Dr. B. Maity, Dr. S.G. Pal, Dr. A. Ghosh, Deptt. of Zoology, Calcutta University who had spared much of their valuable time for interpreting the histopathological slides and ultra-Structural analysis of biological samples.

I am specially indebted to Dr. T.K. Das, Assistant Prof., Deptt. of Anatomy, E.M. facility, A.I.I.M.S., New Delhi for allowing me to avail of the necessary instrumental facilities for ultrastructural analysis of tissue samples.

The active help of Dr. Sushil Chandra Pal, Consulting Physician, Human Genetic Engg. Research Centre, Calcutta, is also acknowledged for chromosomal analysis of samples.

I extend my heartfelt thanks to the Librarian, Chittaranjan National Cancer Institute (CNCI), Calcutta, for her keen interest, encouragement and non-stop help throughout my research work.

Grateful acknowledgements are made to Dr. P.K. Sen, Deptt. of Mathematics, J.U. for his valuable suggestions for statistical analysis of data.

I remain thankful to all the staff of Daya Publishing House, New Delhi for their painstaking work in composing and printing the book in a presentable manner within a short time.

My heartfelt thanks should go to my beloved sister who cheerfully relieved me from most of the family duties and thus made it possible for me to give full attention to research and thereby fulfilling my dreams.

Last but not least, I am indebted to my parents who gave me all their todays for my better tomorrows.

Contents

List of Abbreviations

2-AAF	2-Acetylaminofluorene
AFB_1	Aflatoxin B1
AHH	Aryl hydrocarbon hydroxylase
ATPase	Adenosine triphosphatase
BP	Benzo (a) pyrene
b.p.	Boiling point
BSA	Bovine Serum albumin
CA	Chromosomal aberration
CAM	Cell adhesive molecule
CCl_4	Carbon tetrachloride
CDNB	Chloro-2,4-dinitrobenzene
Cyt-P-450	Cytochrome P-450
C_6H_6	Benzene
$CHCl_3$	Chloroform
DCNB	2,4-dichloronitrobenzene
DDT	1,1-bis (p-chlorophenyl)-2,2, 2-Trichloroethane
DENA	Diethylnitrosamine
DMH	Dimethyl hydrazine
DMN	Dimethylnitrosamine
DNA	Deoxyribonucleic acid
DMBA	7,12-Dimethylbenz(a) anthracene
EM	Electron microscopy
ER	Endoplasmic reticulum
EtOH	Ethanol

$FeCl_3$	Ferric chloride
2-FAA	2 fluorenylacetamide
G-1	Gap between mitosis
G-2	Interval between the end of S phase and the next mitotic division
GPx	Glutathione peroxidase
GSSG	Oxidized glutathione
GGT	γ-glutamyl transpeptidase
G-6-Pase	Glucose-6-phosphatase
GSH	Glutathione
GST	Glutathione S-transferase
G-banding	Giemsa banding
G.I.	Gastro Intestinal tract
GTP	Glutathione S-tranferase placental form
H and E	Haematoxylin and eosin
H.C.C.	Hepatocellular Carcinoma
H.Ns	Hyperplastic nodules
HCl	Hydrochloric acid
IFN	Interferon
ip	intraperitoneal
L	Linn. (author citation)
MDA	Malondialdehyde
M	Mitosis
3′-Met DAB	3′-Methyl-1,4,-dimethylaminoazobenzene
MNU	Methylnitroso urea
NaCl	Sodium Chloride
NaOH	Sodium Hydroxide
NNSP	Non-nodular surrounding parenchyma
PET	Petroleum
P.B	Phenobarbital
PAS	Periodic acid-Schiff

P.C.B.	Polychlorinated biphenyl
ppm	parts per million
PH	Partial hepatectomy
PNs	Persistent nodules
PLC	Primary Liver Cancer
PUFA	Poly unsaturated fatty acid
ROS	Reactive Oxygen Species
S	Synthetic phase
S-180	Sarcoma-180
SAM	Substrate adhesion molecule
SCE	Sister Chromatid exchange
SOD	Superoxide dismutase
TBA	Thiobarbituric acid
TBARS	Thiobarbituric acid reactive substance
TGF-β	Transforming growth factor β
T.P.	Trianthema portulacastrum
TPA	12-0-tetra decanoylphorbol-13-acetate
UDPGA	UDP-glucuronic acid
UDPGT	UDP-glucuronyl transferase
U.S.A.	United States of America
w/w	Weight by weight
w/v	Weight by volume.

1

Introduction

India probably has the oldest and richest cultural tradition in the use of medicinal plants, the first mention of which are in the vedas. About 1,700 plant species are documented comprehensively in Ayurvedic texts for their biological properties, their drug formulations and their effects in a wide range of health conditions varying from the common cold to the different kinds of tumours. Other than Ayurveda there are the Siddha, Unani and Amchi systems of medicine the last being the Tibetian herbal tradition.

There are numerous plant species spread across the length and breadth of India, mostly in the forest areas. A small proportion of these are "lower" plants like lichens, ferns and algae; the majority are from "higher" plant families.

That we take this natural heritage of ours very much for granted is obvious form the current scene. More that 95 per cent of medicinal plant species used by Indian Industry is collected from the wild.

Natural Product Chemists, phytochemists are impressed by the fact that compounds, found in nature, display an unbelievable range of diversity in terms of their structures, physical and biological properties (Wall *et al.*, 1995). These compounds are secondary metabolites with functions in plants, fungi and marine organisms. Currently it is believed that many of these compounds, act in defence of the harmful effects of toxins, Carcinogens or mutagens found in the plant (Mitscher *et al.*, 1986) or attack by external predators. (Woodbury *et al.*, 1961).

During 1950-59 M.E. Wall searched several plants for steroidal saponins, alkaloids, tanins, sterols, flavonoids etc. (Wall *et al.*, 1954a,b; Wall *et al.*, 1957; Wall *et al.*, 1961). The survey included not only quantitative data but also qualitative analysis. Plant collection was done by botanists under the auspices of the plant introduction division of USDA. After screening, the plants were subjected to tests for antitumour, antibiotic and antiviral activity.

1. Anticancer Plants

Several plants have been screened throughout the world for anticancer activities. *Cryptoporus volvatus* was extracted by Kim Byong, Robberts James E., Purdue University. U.S.A. (1982). The antitumour fraction is a protein-polysaccharide complex, containing 18.2% protein, 55.3% polysaccharide. The fraction was tested with sarcoma 180, implanted in A-strain mice. Turnover inhibition ratio was 80.4% for high doses and 70.3% for low doses. Takemoto T. *et al.* (1983) isolated Pfaffic acid, a novel nortriterpene and its monoacetate Meester from *Pfaffia paniculata* kuntze. The compound showed high inhibitory effects on the growth of cultured tumour cells i.e. He La (s-3), Melanoma B-16, and lewis lung Carcinoma cells at 4-6 mg/ml.

Fractionation of an aqueous EtOH extract of the wood of *Simba multiflora,* afforded a new antineoplastic quassinoid 6a Senecioyloxy chapparin, in addition to two known quassinoids– Chaparrinone and 6a senecioloxy–chapparrinone. (Arisawa *et al.*, 1983) which displayed activity against KB and P-388 test systems Table 1.1. The antitumour alkaloid 11-hydroxy-20(s) Camptothecin (I) was isolated from the woody tissue of *Camptotheca acuminata.* It displayed marked antitumour activity against L 1210 Leukaemia in mice. There was no toxic effect observed even at relatively high doses (Wall *et al.*, 1986).

Micromimutin–a novel cytotoxic coumarin from *Micromelum minutum* displayed strong cytotoxic activities. (Tantivatana, 1983). There was the co-occurrence of the epoxide phebalosin, in the same plant. Phebalosin was toxic to brine shrimp (LC_{50} 47 ppm) and was inhibitory to the development of crown gall tumours on potatoe discs (-64% and -70%) in 2 independent determinations.

Table 1.1 : Anti-tumour, Anti-cancer, Anti-leukaemic Plants of the World and Their Active Constituents

Botanical name of plant	*Plant part used*	*Therapeutic value*	*Active component*
1. *Cryptoporus volvatus*	'Carpo-phores'	Anti-tumour activity against sarcoma 180	Protein-polysaccharide complex
2. *Pffafia paniculata*	Roots	Active against Melanoma B-16 HeLa S-3 etc.	Pfaffic acid
3. *Simba multiflora*	Wood	Activity against KB, P-388 system	Quassinoid
4. *Camptotheca acuminata*	Wood	Against L-1210 leukaemia in animal models	Camptothesin (I)
5. *Helianthus annus*	Leaves	Active against Ehrlrich's carcinoma	Germacranolide
6. *Murraya Koenign*	Root, bark	Cytotoxic against KB cell line	Koenoline
7. *Nicandra physalodes*	Root, bark	Cytotoxic	Withanolide, Nicandenone
8. *Polyporus versicolor*	Whole plant	Active against rat hepatoma cells	Steroids
9. *Curcuma xanthorhiza*	Rhizome	Active against sarcoma 180	Sesquiterpenoids
10. *Pterocarpus indicus*	Bark	Carcinostatic effect on sarcoma 180	Bioactive poly-phenolic compounds
11. *Dracena afromontana*	Twigs	Cytotoxic to KB cells	Afromontoxide (I)
12. *Gutierrezia resinosa*	Twigs	Active against human carcinoma of nasopharynx	Flavones I and II
13. *Brucea antidysentria*	Fruits	Antitumor activity	Quassinoids, alkaloids
14. *Crinum asiaticum*	Fruits	Cytotoxic activity	Alkaloids
15. *Psorospermum febrifugum*	Root	Active against P-388 system	Xanthone Psorospermin
16. *Mallotus japonicus*	Pericarp	Cytotoxic	Mallatophenone (I) mallatochrome (II)
17. *Cicuta maculata*	Whole plant	Anti leukaemic	Cicultoxin

Insignificant cytotoxic activity was observed in case of 9 ASK astrocytoma reversal assay. (Tantishaiyakul *et al.*, 1986).

Annuithrin (I) a biologically active germacranolide, isolated from the young leaves of *Helianthus annus*. Annuithrin I was found to be a growth inhibitor in straight growth test and antibacterial tests. It inhibited the synthesis of DNA/RNA in cells of ascites form of Ehrlich's carcinoma (Otmar *et al.*, 1981).

Carpophores of *Ganoderma lucidum*, a species of Korean basidiomycetean fungus, showed marked antitumour activity against sarcoma 180, at doses of 50 mg/kg/day for 10 days. The tumour inhibition was 87.6% and the tumours in 5 of the 15 mice were completely regressed. The antitumor fraction, consisted of a complex of polysaccharide protein, in which 4 monosaccharides and 18 amino acids were identified (Kak *et al.*, 1980).

Ganoderic acids T and Z, 2 cytotoxic triterpenes were isolated from the same fungus. Ganoderic acids showed in vitro cytotoxic activities against hepatoma cells (Jorgeo *et al.*, 1983). Crude extracts of the European wood rotting fungus *Polyporus versiolor* contains Cytotoxic metabolites. These were found to be cytotoxic to rat hepatoma cells (Valisolalao *et al.*, 1983).

Bisabolane sesquiterpenoids from *Curcuma xanthorrhiza* revealed marked antitumor effects. The active components α-Curcumene, ar-turmerone, β-atlantone and Xanthorrhizol were very active against Sarcoma 180; ascites in mice (Itokawa *et al.*, 1985).

Bio-active polyphenolic constituents from the bark of *Pterocarpus indicus* had carcinostatic effect on mice with Ehrlich's carcinoma at a dose of 2 mg/kg body weight of the animals (Takeuchi *et al.*, 1986). The substance also displayed remarkable plasmin esterolytic activity at ED_{50}=2.5 μg/ml.

Biologically active flavones from *Guterrezia resinosa*, showed significant activities against human carcinoma of the nasopharynx (Biltner *et al.*, 1983).

Hispidulin – a cytotoxic flavone from *Centaurea urvillei* leaves, showed cytotoxicity at 0.05 mg/ml in L-Strain fibroblasts (Ulubelen *et al.*, 1982).

Crinafoline (I), Crinafolidine (II) isolated from *Crinum latifolium* brought about significant reduction in the viability and in-vivo growth of S-180 ascites tumour cells (Ghoshal *et al.*, 1986).

An antitumour glucan (HA-b Glucan) was isolated from the neutral polysaccharide fraction of a hot water extract of the edible mushroom *Pleurotus ostreatus*. Purification was accomplished by extraction with 20% NaCl solution saturated with thymol and by precipitation with EtOH and DMSO solutions. The glucan showed remarkable antitumour activity at a dose of 0.1 mg/kg body weight (Yoshiyoka *et al.*, 1985).

Lapachol, 2-isopropenylfurano-1,4 = napthoquinone (I) and dehydro a-lapachone were isolated from the C_6H_6 extract of *Markhamia hildebrandti*. A laboratory experiment on tissue culture, showed that (I) is a powerful antitumour agent, active against He La cells. The concentration for inhibiting 50% growth (ID_{50}) of HeLa cells was 7.5×10^{-7} M (Cheng *et al.*, 1986). Proflamin – a biological response modifying antitumour agent was isolated from the culture mycelium of *Flammulina velutipes* by ion exchange column chromatography and molecular sieving. The antitumour effect of Proflamin was studied with murine tumours. It was markedly effective against syngenic tumours, B-16 melanoma and adenocarcinoma 755. Proflamin exhibited no cytocidal effect against cultured cell-lines *in vitro*. Oral administration of Proflamin produced no lethal or adverse effect in mice (Ikikawa *et al.*, 1985).

Cytotoxic diterpenes – a new ring A secotriterpene koetjapic acid (I) and 30×0-olean-12 en -29oic-acid, katonic acid (II), and some others, spathulenol and caryophyllene were isolated from the stems of *Sanodoricum koetjape*. Both I and II showed Cytotoxic activity against a variety of cultured human cancer cells (Kaneda *et al.*, 1992).

A variety of phloroglucinol derivatives were isolated from the pericarps of *Mallotus japonicus*. They were assessed for growth inhibiting activity against human larynx (HE_p-2) and Lung (PC-13) carcinoma cells as well as mouse B 16 melanoma, and L 5178Y cells. They were significantly cytotoxic in culture. (Arisawa *et al.*, 1990). Antitumour constituents -3, (3.3 dimethylallyl)-5-(-3-acetyl-2,-4-dihydroxy-5-methyl-6-methoxybenzyl)-phloracetophenone displayed marked cytotoxic activity against all target tumour cells and produced marked prolongation of life span in mice bearing L 5178Y Leukaemia. 22-hydroxytingenone isolated from the same plant *Glyptopetalum sclerocarpum* also showed intense cytotoxic activity against KB carcinoma of nasopharynx, col-2 colon cancer.

HT 1080 fibrosarcoma, BC-1 breast cancer and MEL-2 melanoma (Bavovada *et al.*, 1990) Cytotoxic polyketides-10,13 trans-13,14 erythrodensicoumarin (I), 10,13, trans, 13, 14, threodensicoumarin (II), 8-hydroxy annoracin from the stem bark of *Annona densicoma* were active against lung carcinoma (A-549), Colon adenocarcinoma (HT-29) cell lines with ED_{50} of 4.10^{-4} and 1×10^{-5} mg.ml (Jing *et al.*, 1992).

Funoran, an algal polysaccharide from *Gloiopeltis tenax*, significantly inhibited the growth of Ehrlich ascites carcinoma and solid Ehrlih Meth-A-fibrosarcoma and sarcoma 180 tumours. In tumour bearing mice, funoran significantly induced the enhancement of delayed type hypersensitivity response to sheep R.B.C. The antitumour effect of funoran is related to augmentation of T-helper, T-Cytotoxic and NK cells (Ren *et al.*, 1995).

Phenanthrenes-4,7-dihydroxy-2-methoxy-9,10-dihydrophenan threne (I) and Denbinobin (II) from the aerial parts of *Dendrobium nobile* were cytotoxic against A 549 (human lung carcinoma), SK-OV-3 (human ovary adeno-carcinoma and other cell lines. (I) displayed antitumour activity on the life span of ICR mice intraperitonially implanted with 1×10^{6} cells of sarcoma 180 (Lee *et al.*, 1995).

The amaryllidaceae alkaloids pretazettine, was highly cytotoxic to Molt 4 Lymphoid cells. Lycoreminine was highly cytotoxic against HepG-2 hepatoma cells. Both showed fibroblastic activity against LMTK cells. (Wenger *et al.*, 1995).

Four Cytotoxic lignans–Deoxypodophyllotoxin (I), b-peltatin-methylether(II), Picro b-peltatin methyl-ether (III) and dehydro b-Peltatin methyl ether, isolated from the stem bark of *Bursera permollis*, were found to be potentially cytotoxic when evaluated against a panel of human cancer cell lines (Wickramaratne *et al.*, 1995) Table 1.2, Fig. 1.1.

In 1988, the remarkable clinical efficacy of taxol resulted in numerous observations of partial and complete remission of advanced ovarian cancer in women and move recently there are reports of the efficacy of the drug in breast lung and prostrate cancer (Wall *et al.*, 1967; Wani *et al.*, 1971). Early studies with crude extracts revealed activity against walker tumour inhibition assay and modest activity in L 1210 Leukaemia and particularly high activity in 1534 (P4) Leukaemia assay, SRC Cx-1 colon xenograft; SRC Lx-1 lungxenograft and SRC Mx-1 mammary xenograft in

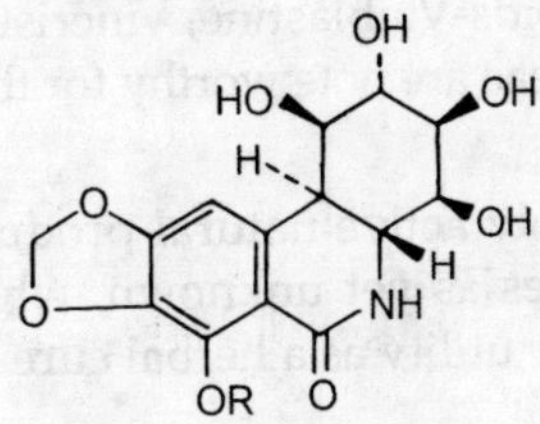

A. Structure of 'Pancratisatin' isolated from *P. littorale*

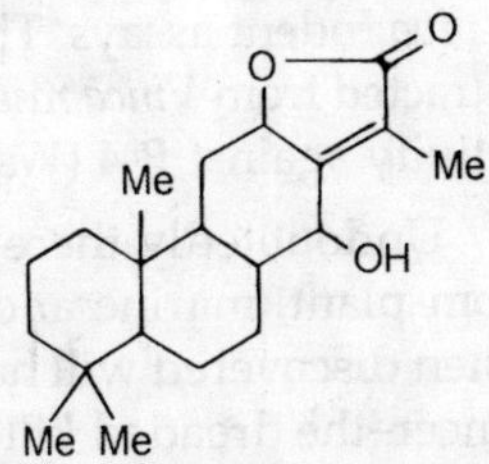

B. Structure of 'Triaculetin-I' isolated from *E. triculeata*

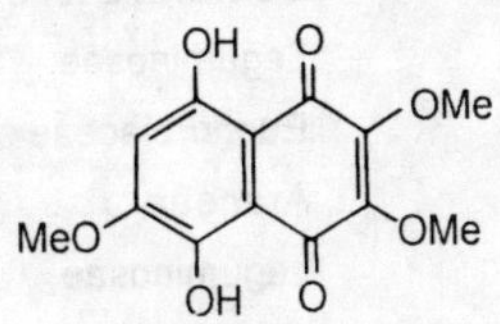

C. Structure of 'Trichozani B' isolated from *T. crocosmaeflora*

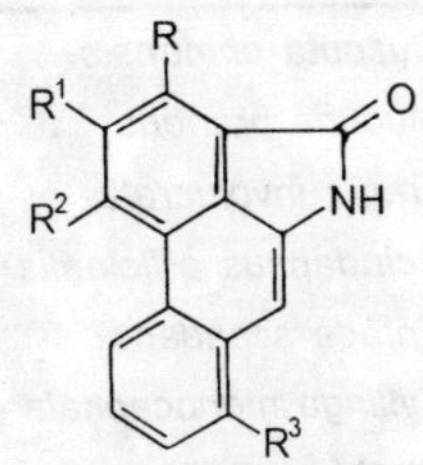

D. Structure of 'Aristolactam I' isolated from *P. flos-avis*

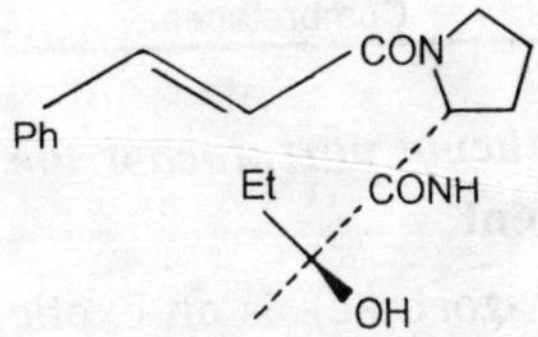

E Structure of (–) – odorinol diamide from *A. odorata*

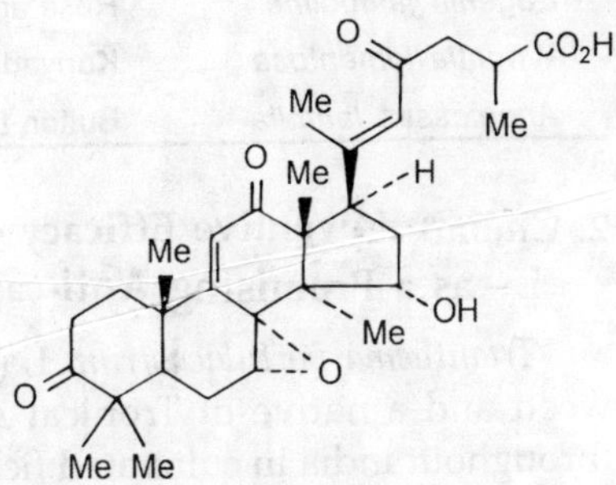

F. Structure of Applanoxidic acid from *G. applanatum*

Fig. 1.1 : Structures of Some Compounds Exhibiting Anti-neoplastic Effects.

in vivo rodent assays. The Vinca alkaloids-Vinblastine, Vincristine extracted from *Vinca rosea* of Apocynaceae are note worthy for their activity against P-4 (Wall *et al.*, 1995).

Undoubtedly there are other highly active natural products from plant, marine and fungal sources as yet unknown, which when discovered will have therapeutic utility as a herbal cure for cancer–the dreaded killer disease.

Table 1.2 : Anticancer Plants – Ethnobotanical Survey, India

Name	*Common Name/ Local Name*	*Family*
Cuscuta chinensis	Swarnalata	Convolvulaceae
Mucuna pruriens	Alkushi	Leguminosae
Tragia involucrata	Nettle	Euphorbiaceae
Scindapsus officinalis	Gajpipal	Araceae
Entada scandens	Gila	Leguminosae
Kyllinga monocephala	Swetgodhubi	Cyperaceae
Streblus asper	Sehora	Moraceae
Gloriosa superba	Agnishikha	Liliaceae
Viscum attenuatum	Mistletoe	Loranthaceae
Eugenia jambolina	Rose apple	Myrtaceae
Wrightia tomentosa	Koriyadudh	Apocynaceae
Anogiessus latifolia	Button tree	Combretaceae

2. Chemo Preventive Efficacy of *Trianthema portulacastrum* L – as a Promising Anti-cancer Agent

Trianthema portulacastrum L (family Aizoaceae), is an exotic weed and a native of Tropical America. It is now naturalized throughout India in cultivated fields, river beds, waste places etc. (Chatterjee *et al.*, 1994). The plant is a diffuse prostrate, glabrous, succulent herb with angular much branched stems (Kirtikar *et al.*, 1975; Chatterjee *et al.*, 1994). Flowers are pink, white, solitary, apical in position (Chadha *et al.*, 1976).

The chemical composition of the whole plant of *T. Portulacastrum* indicates moisture 91.3, protein, 2, fat 0.4, carbohydrate 3.2, crude fibre 0.9 and ash 2.2 gm; calcium 100, Phosphorus 30, Iron 38.5, Ascorbic acid 70 mgs per 100 gm, carotine 2.3 mg per 100 gm (Chadha *et al.*, 1976). The crude protein content of *Triánthema* is comparable with many of the rich legume fodders like berseem, lucerne, cowpea (Sen *et al.*, 1978). Chemical analysis of the weed indicates its potential value as a source of organic matter to the soil. It enriches the soil with nitrogen, phosphorus and potassium (Mudaliar and Rao, 1958).

T. portulacastrum contains an alkaloid Trianthemine $C_{32}H_{46}O_6N_2$; $_{mp}$127°C (Chadha *et al.*, 1976; Chatterjee *et al.*, 1994). It contains Ecdysterone, the most widely occurring phytoecdysone. This has been reported to act as a chemosterilant and is also known to possess moulting hormone activity. Ecdysterone gave full pupation-response for larvae of housefly (Banerji *et al.*, 1971). *T. portulacastrum* is known to contain straight and branched chain alkanes (Singh *et al.*, 1982a). High levels of oxalic acid, betacyanin and 3, 4-dimethoxycinnamic acid have been isolated from plant samples (Bharadwaj *et al.*, 1987; Bharadwaj *et al.*, 1988; Ravishankar *et al.*, 1979; Singh *et al.*, 1982b). Detectable levels of quercetin and ferulic acid is reported to build up during stress, produced by fungal infection (Parikh *et al.*, 1992). Recently flavonoids and other related compounds, with potent agrochemical activity, were isolated. *T. portulacastrum* contains a bioflavonoid leptorumol. In addition longchain alcohols, -sitosterol, stigmasterol and their β-glucopyranosides have been isolated (Kokpol *et al.*, 1997).

The plant has been found to be efficacious in the therapy of a broad spectrum of ailments (Chopra *et al.*, 1959; Kirtiker *et al.*, 1975). It is an important medicinal plant, used in Ayurvedic and Unani systems of medicine (Fazal *et al.*, 1978; Vohra *et al.*, 1983). The plant is attributed with analgesic, stomachic, ulcerative, inflammatory and abortifacient properties (Kirtikar *et al.*, 1975; Singh *et al.*, 1983). The root is cathartic, abortifacient with irritant properties. An infusion of the roots is administered in jaundice, stranguary and dropsy. A decoction of the herb is a vermifuge, useful in rheumatism. It is said to be antidotal to alcoholic poison. (Chadha *et al.*, 1976; Chatterjee *et al.*, 1994). *Trianthema portulacastrum* Linn has proved to be extremely valuable in the treatment of asthma, bronchitis, ascites, cardiovascular disorder, migraine etc (Chopra *et al.*, 1958; Wahid *et al.*, 1961; Nayar *et al.*, 1980). Crude extracts from roots and leaves have been reported to exert general Pharmacodynamic and antifertility effects (Jamwal *et al.*, 1962; Gupta *et al.*, 1976; Garg *et al.*, 1976).

Recently our laboratory has documented, a marked antihepatotoxic acitivity of an EtOH fraction of the whole plant (excluding roots) against acute hepatocellular injury induced by alcohol and Carbontetrachloride in mice (Bishayee *et al.*, 1996).

In CCl_4 induced chronic liver damage in mice, the beneficial response of the extract has been well reflected in the normalization of altered serum transaminases, as well as enzymes of plasma membrane, microsomal, Lysosomal and Cytoplasmic fractions of hepatic tissue (Mandal *et al.*, 1997).

All these studies and also those carried out elsewhere made it worth-while to look for its chemopreventive role in a defined experimental Carcinogenesis model. However the real anticarcinogenic potential of this plant against a more sophisticated system of experimentally induced carcinogenesis needs to be evaluated. Further the plant with its diversified biochemical and pharmacological activities may be a valuable therapeutic agent in the near future for combatting the killer disease cancer.

3. Cancer

3.1 Terminology

The terms Cancer and Carcinoma appear to have the same origin (L. Cancer means Crab, GK Karkinos; Sans Karakarata). The Clawlike venous pattern and tenacious malignant tumours, suggested to the ancient people, the analogy between Crab and Cancer (Kothari and Mehta, 1972).

3.2 The Cancerous State

Cancer has largely been viewed as a cellular disease. The macroscopic tumour represents a large population of similar cells, sharing a common set of genetic aberrations. A special terminology has grown up for cells in culture. Cells are said to be transformed when they show certain permnent abnormalities (Porten, 1974). 3 operationally distinct forms of transformation are associated with the cancerous state.

Normal cells never exhibit any of the listed transformations. Cellular adhesive property and substrate environment are crucial to morphogenesis and organogenesis. From the initial stages of embriyonic development altered adhesive properties often lead to disease states.

Table 1.3 : The Characteristics of the Cancerous State

Type of Alteration	*Symptoms*	*Essential features*
I. Irregular growth transformation	Lack of contact inhibition	Failure of intercellular contact to paralyse cell-membrane motion (i.e. persisting activity of lamellipodia)
II. Unrestrained growth transformation	Lack of density dependent inhibition of cell multiplication	Persisting proliferation in densely concentrated cell population. (increased terminal cell density)
III. Infinite growth transformation.	Establishment of a permanent cell line.	Capacity of cells to undergo an infinite number of divisions.

Cell-cell adhesion and cell substrate adhesion are mediated by 2 major categories of molecules–cell adhesive molecules (CAMs) and cell substrate adhesion molecules (SAMs). The interplay of CAM's and SAM's is vital to a number of normal and pathological phenomena, such as neurite outgrowth and targeting, lymphocyte homing and infiltration, bone repairs, tissue regeneration and metastasis of tumour cells (Brodt, 1996).

Cancer is a disease marked by UN-controlled proliferation of cells, with the resultant production of contagious cellular masses–the tumours. The cells thus divide anarchically giving rise to a large mass of new tissue–the neoplasm (Constantinides, 1984) Cancerous cells lose their specialisation and spread from the tumour through out the blood stream, into the lymphatics by a process called metastasis and new growths may form in other parts of the body. The following characteristics are essentially observed in a cancer cell.

- Immortalisation – i.e. possibility of a theoretically unlimited number of divisions.
- "Transformation" which is manifested by
  - loss of contact inhibition.
  - loss of need to anchor.
- Agglutinability – they develop new surface antigens and more lectin receptors in their carbohydrate coat.

- Display structural and chemical anaplasia.
- Grow into malignant tumours when transplanted into syngenic or immunosuppressed animals.

Cancer cells show profound biological abnormality when they interact with their surroundings. They exhibit non-responsiveness to extra-cellular growth inhibitory signals. Traits of mitogen independence and refractoriness to growth represent a part of complex biology of cancer cells.

It is now known from studies conducted by Hunt, 1991; Motokuna, 1991; Hartwell, 1992; that a cell-cycle clock exists. It represents the ultimate recipient of all positive and negative signals, that influence cell proliferation. All the circuits that control cell growth must eventually feed into and affect the cell-cycle clock. The actions of oncogenes and tumour suppressor proteins must ultimately be understood in terms of how they influence the workings of a cell-cycle clock (EL-Deiry *et al.*, 1993; Makela *et al.*, 1994). The connection forged to date between oncogenes, tumour suppressor genes and the clock are still tenuous or non existent.

3.3 *Normal and Abnormal Growth Control*

In the post-fertilization phase, the dividing embriyonic cells initiate a multifaceted programme of cellular differentiation. There is stringent regulation over cell proliferation. In adult organisms, some cells fail to proliferate, others become terminally differentiated and lose power to divide, still others divide only when replacement becomes necessary. A cell that disobeys the normal contraints on proliferation, gives rise to a tumour.

3.4 *Normal Growth Control*

The cellular environment and state of differentiation exerts regulatory influence on cell proliferation. The environment supplies positive stimulatory signals and negative inhibitory signals. The balance between both these types of signals regulates the growth, development and maintenance of complex tissues and organs. The state of differentiation dictates, as to how a cell should respond to a particular signal. Cell proliferation takes place after an orderly progression of biochemical and cellular events. Cells in the proliferating stage divide into two daughter cells.

In actively dividing cells, the gap between cell divisions is represented by the cell cycle. The cell cycle is subdivided into four distinct spaces, separated in time–Mitosis (M) $G_1S_1G_2$. G_1 represents the interval between the end of mitosis and beginning of DNA replication (S). G_2 is the interval between the ends of the "S" or synthetic phase and initiation of the next mitotic division. Length of cell cycle is variable and in mammals it can be as short as 10 hours or as long as several days.

Cell proliferation is controlled by positive as well as negative regulatory mechanisms and influences growth state transitions and progress through the cell cycle. Neoplastic growth is due to increased sensitivity to or activation of growth stimulatory mechanisms or from decreased sensitivity to or inactivation of growth inhibitory mechanism (Marx, 1986).

Like growth, stimulation is very often mediated by environmental factors, that have the ability to change/modify the expression of growth related genes. Many growth inhibitory factors are tissue/cell specific eg. Polypeptide transforming growth factor β (TGF-β) reversibly inhibits epithelial cell proliferation but stimulates anchorage-independent growth of many fibroblasts. On the other hand Interferons–a class of virus coded gene proteins can inhibit reversibly the growth of a number of cell-types (Ford and Maizel, 1984).

There are however, other genes, whose products act intracellularly to suppress cell proliferation (Marx, 1986). These are designated as antiproliferative or suppressor genes. Much is still unknown about the exact mechanism by which such genes may act.

3.5 *Abnormal Growth Control*

Tumour cells exhibit similar patterns as that of normal cells, in that they like normal cells, pass through all four phases of the cell cycle, when they proliferate. Tumour cells are defective in one or more regulatory mechanisms that usually checks inappropriate proliferation. In addition tumour cells modify the local environment in such a manner as to make it conducive for cell proliferation. These changes are due to one or more mutations in the tumour cell DNA.

Tumour cells from different sources display a wide range of growth control defects. The relaxed control exhibited by tumour cells, results from increased sensitivity to positive signals or decreased sensitivity to negative signals. There is enough evidence that no single derangement in growth control can fully account for the neoplastic phenotype. So by the time a tumour is detected, the cells have already undergone multiple changes, that allows autonomous proliferation (Weinberg, 1985). The existence of multiple growth control points only tends to ensure that uncontrolled proliferation is a relatively rare occurrence. Prevention and cure of Cancer needs a deeper understanding of the molecular mechanisms that regulates proliferation of normal cells and the mechanisms by while tumour cells overcome these controls.

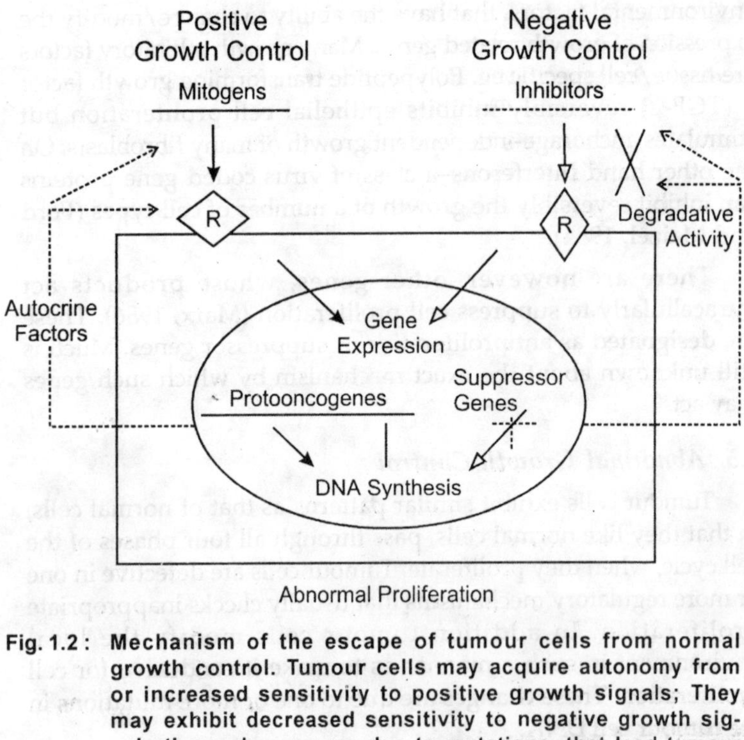

Fig. 1.2 : Mechanism of the escape of tumour cells from normal growth control. Tumour cells may acquire autonomy from or increased sensitivity to positive growth signals; They may exhibit decreased sensitivity to negative growth signals these changes are due to mutations, that lead tumour cells to modify their environment, that activates proto oncogenes or inactivate supressorgenes.

R = receptor.

Table 1.4 : Cell Transformation - Properties

I. On growth and cell division

(a) High saturation density.
(b) Loss of contact inhibition.
(c) Immortality.
(d) Low serum requirement.
(e) Growth factor independence.
(f) Growth in immune-deficient animals.
(g) Anchorage independence.

II. Plasma membrane related changes

(a) Changes in agglutinability.
(b) Inability of actin filaments to organize properly.
(c) Increased nutrient transport.
(d) Decreased quantities of surface and extracellular fibronectin.
(e) Increased secretion of plasminogen activator.

III. Oncogene activation

(a) Over expression of ras-gene.
(b) Point mutation in ras-gene.
(c) Cooperativity of myc and ras.

4. Carcinogenesis : From Animal Models to Molecular Models in One Decade

Carcinogenesis is a general term used to denote the development of neoplasia. It is a phenomenon induced by a variety of agents-chemical, physical, biological and genetic (Pitot, 1987). Table 1.5 denotes representative examples of each type of carcinogenic agent, and range of their molecular masses in daltons (Table 1.5).

In both biological and genetic carcinogenesis, the carcinogenic agent, consists of informational macromolecules, either DNA or RNA of high molecular weights on the other hand radiation carcinogenesis may not result from the action of informational macromolecules, but rather from the direct (Haseltine, 1983) or indirect (Biaglow, 1981) action of high energy photons, or particles with existing DNA. Carcinogenesis by small molecular weight chemicals, involves either a direct action of the chemical on cellular DNA or metabolism of the parent chemical to an active or ultimate form, which can then react with cellular DNA to produce a permanent chemical change in the DNA structure (Pitot, 1986a).

There are several other instances in chemical carcinogenisis where induction of carcinogenisis does not directly involve structural modification of DNA (Ashby and Tennant, 1988) (Table 1.6).

Table 1.5 : Categories of Carcinogenic agents

Class	*Example*	*Relative molecular mass (in daltons)*
I. Chemical	Poly-cyclic hydrocarbons, aromatic amines, halides, diet, hormone, metals and polymer surface.	$5 \times 10^1 – 5 \times 10^4$
II. Radiation	Ionizing (X and Y ray, particle radition) uv raditions, (UVA, UVB)	$<<<1 – 1^+$
III. Biological	Viruses, (Papova, Herpes, Retro, Hepadnoviruses)	3×10^6-170×10^6 (viral genomes)
IV. Genetic	Transgenesis by Enhancer Promoter, oncogene constitutents and selective breeding.	$\sim 10^6 – 10^8$

Table 1.6 : Carcinogenic Agents or Processes Incapable of Inducing Direct Structural Changes

A	:	Polypeptides and Steroid hormones.
B	:	Inert substances, Plastic film Carcinogenesis.
C	:	Alcoholic beverages, ethanol.
D	:	Specific dietary alterations. (Methyl deficiency, galactosamine excess)
E	:	Chemicals with no DNA reactive intermediates.
F	:	Calorie intake.

Some agents are able to induce structural changes in the DNA molecule, without evidence that they are carcinogenic (Shelby and Stasiwicz, 1984). So it is not possible to develop a general mechanism of carcinogenesis, that is applicable to all carcinogenic agents (Pitot and Dragan, 1991). On the other hand, a reconciliation of the disparate actions of carcinogenic agents, with a general process of carcinogenesis may be viewed differently in the light of our increased understanding of the natural history of the pathogenesis of neoplasia.

4.1 Multistage Carcinogenesis

During the last decade, chemical carcinogenesis research has broadened our understanding of the cellular and molecular changes involved in cancer development and led to the identification of stages in the entire process. Neoplasia is preceded by a latent period from the time of first administration of a carcinogenic agent to the development of visible neoplastic lesions. Our initial understanding of the biological events, occurring during the latency period of neoplasia was pioneered during early 1940's, by several workers studying epidermal carcinogenesis in mouse model (Rous and Kidd, 1941; Berenblum and Shubik, 1947). From these studies 2 stages of the latent period could be identified. They are initiation and promotion. Foulds (1954) working on mammary adenocarcinoma of mouse, modified the concept of the stage of promotion; to include all events after initiation, and used the term progression to refer to all post-initiation events in neoplastic development. So at least 2 stages- Promotion and Progression follow the stage of initiation. This demarcation was partly due to the use of carcinogenic protocols different from those of original experiments of 1940's and 1950's (Potter, 1981; Hennings and Yuspa, 1985). Multistage carcinogenesis has also been demonstrated during carcinogenesis in a variety of different tissues in the past decades (Pitot, 1986a). The typical features of initiation, promotion and progression are depicted in Table 1.7.

Table 1.7 : Stages of Carcinogenesis Features

Stage	Features
A : Initiation	Irreversible, needs fixation, additive without threshold.
B : Promotion	Reversible, environmentally modulated, maximal response threshold.
C : Progression	Irreversible somatic, aneuploidy, progressive karyotypic instability.

4.2 Initiation

Initiation takes place first in the natural history of neoplastic develoment and reflects a permanent irreversible change in the initiated cells (Boutwell, 1964). It involves exposure of normal cells to chemical, physical or microbial carcinogens that produce genetic changes, and provide initiated cells with altered responsiveness to the micro environment on one hand and on the other hand it exerts a selective clonal expansion advantage, compared to normal surrounding cells (Yuspa and Harris, 1982). Initiated cells have decreased responsiveness to inter and intracellular signals and maintain normal tissue architecture and regulate homeostatic growth and maturation of cells. Initiated cells are less responsive to negative growth factors, inducers of terminal cell differentiation and/or programmed cell death-apoptosis (Yuspa and Poirier, 1988; Moses *et al.*, 1990; Rotello *et al.*, 1991). Efficiency of initiation is related to cellular replicative DNA systhesis and cell division (Ishikawa, 1980). DNA synthesis is needed for fixation and so there is irreversibility of initiated cells (Mc Cornick and Bertram, 1982).

4.3 Promotion

Promotion leads to the proliferation and/or suvival of initiated cells to a greater extent than normal cells and serves to enhance the probability of additional genetic damage including endogenous mutations, which accumulates in the expanding population of these cells. The probability of a sub-population of initiated cells, converting to malignancy, can be substantially increased by further exposure to DNA damaging agents. (Hennings, 1989) that may activate protooncogenes (Yuspa *et al.*, 1990) and/or inactivate tumour suppressor genes. This stage is characterized by its operational reversibility. Promotion is modulated by various environmental factors, including the frequency with which the promoting agent is administered (Wattenberg, 1978), age of the test animal, (Van Duuren, 1975) composition and amount of diet, (Wattenberg, 1978; Sargent *et al.*, 1989). Promoters exhibit threshold or no effect level as well as maximum response. The relative potency of promoting agents is determined in multistage hepatocarcinogensis in rat (Pitot *et al.*, 1987). Since promoters exhibit a threshhold, and show reversibility they have low risk for induction of cancer if the dose and frequency of exposure are low.

4.4 Progression

Progression is generally marked by karyotypic instability, and evolution and further development of irreversible, aneuploid malignant neoplasias. This is a major point of distinction between progression and other events i.e. initiation and promotion. Such alterations in the structure of the genome of the neoplastic cell, during this stage are directly related to the increased growth rate, invasiveness, metastatic capability, and biochemical changes in the malignant cell. These changes, as reflections of karyotypic alterations, continue to evolve during the stage of progression, in a variety of different neoplasms, such as multistage epidermal carcinogenesis (Aldaz *et al.*, 1987) leukaemia and lymphoma (Nowell, 1986) and multistage hepatocarcinogenesis (Sargent *et al.*, 1989). Irreversibility of progression has been assumed. Environmental alterations frequently produce changes in gene expression, growth rate and functional processes within cells during progression (Noble, 1977; Horsfall *et al.*, 1986). Progessor agents must be capable of inducing genetic damage typical of progression. Such agents should include clastrogens and complete carcinogens i.e. agents capable of inducing malignant transformation from initiation through progression.

It is likely that transcriptional and/or mutational activation of proto and cellular oncogenes, growth factors, nuclear DNA binding proteins, and other unknown cellular oncogenes may occur easily during progression and become mechanistically associated with its development. Since karyotypic changes is one major mechanism that can induce both transcriptional and mutational activation of protooncogenes, karyotypic instability becomes the common denominator for the genesis and maintenance of the stage of progression.

Multistage carcinogenesis mediated by the agents is tabled (Table 1.8).

4.5 Cell and Molecular Mechanisms in Chemical Carcinogenesis–Classification of Chemical Carcinogens

The expression of varied biological effects of chemical carcinogens, depend upon their interaction with cell constituents. This occurs via covalent reactions that leads to the formation of carcinogen adducts (Cooper *et al.*, 1995).

In some cases carcinogens may be spontaneously reactive in biological media, but for most part, they are inert and require conversion to a reactive intermediate. Mixed function oxidases convert xenobiotics to highly reactive electrophillic agents that reacts instantly with nucleophilic sites in the substrate molecules (Miller, 1978).

Table 1.8 : Multistage Carcinogenesis-Agents

I. Initiator	:	Brings about initiation of cells only.
II. Promoter	:	Brings about reversible expansion of initiated cell clones eg. UVA radiation.
III. Progressor	:	Converts initiated cells/cell in promotion phase to a potentially malignant cell.
IV. Complete Carcinogen	:	Can induce cancer in normal cells having the combined properties of initiation, promotion, progression.

Chemical carcinogens are classified according to the chemical group to which they belong eg : polynuclear aromatic hydrocarbons, aromatic amines, alkylating agents including N-Nitrosocompounds. DNA has become universally recognized as a critical target for the action of carcinogens. Studies on the mechanism of carcinogen action have focussed upon the role of DNA adducts and their ability to introduce heritable changes in DNA (Cooper *et al.*, 1995). The alkylating agents as a group of nitroso compounds in particular have attracted attention because of their ubiquity in human environment (Bartsch and Montesano, 1984).

Further due to the simple nature of the adducts, formed in the substrate molecules, they confer better long term prospects for understanding their role at the molecular level. O^6-genomic alkylation is most studied (Lijinsky, 1995). Effects commonly envcountered as a result of exposure to alkylating agents include toxicity, mutagenesis, clastrogenesis, transformation, carcinogenesis, teratogenesis and other transplacental effects. (Marquison and O' connor, 1990).

The stages of carcinogenesis induced by agents is tabled (Table 1.9).

5. Experimental Hepatocarcinogenesis : An Overview

Several models of hepatocarcinogenesis have been proposed (Reuber, 1965; Epstein, 1967; Becker, 1978; Solt and Farber, 1976; Solt, 1977; Farber, 1980; Sells, 1979; Shinozuka, 1979; Columbano, 1982; Rao, 1983; Farber, 1984a). The liver has currently shot into the limelight, as a suitable target for chemical carcinogenesis, ever since Sasaki and Yoshida (1935) described the carcinoma induced by butter yellow in rats. Since then experimental hepatic tumours have become a favourite model for investigating carcinogenesis. Various chemicals of diverse nature (Miller and Miller, 1976a, Miller, 1978), radiations, (Curtis and Tilley, 1972) and few viruses, (Stenback *et al.*, 1973; Lapis *et al.*, 1975) have been implicated in the development of experimental liver cancer in several species. Various chemicals and hormones also play a role (Goldfarb, 1976; Sherlock 1979). Hepatitis B virus (Blumberg, 1977; Zuckerman, 1978) can induce liver cancer in human beings.

Table 1.9 : Stages of Carcinogenesis Induced by Specific Agents

Class of Compounds	*Example*	*Stage/Stages*
I	Diethylnitrosoamine, aflatoxin B1, Uretane, 2-acetylaminofluorene tobacco smoke	Initiation, Promotion, Progression
	Phenobarbital, Tetradecanoyl-Phorbol acetate, dietary fat, ethanol	Promotion, Progression
	Prolactin, Oestrogen, androgen	Promotion
	Foreign body, asbestos, benzene, Potassium arsenite	Progression
II	Ionizing radiation (UVB, UVC)	Initiation and Progression
	UVA radiation	Promotion
III	Papova, retro, Epstein-Bar viruses	Progression
	Herpes and Hepadina Virus	Progression
IV	Transgenesis	Promotion, Progression
	Selective breeding	Initiation Promotion, Progression

The liver is a frequent site for the development of chemically induced cancer in rodents. This is because the liver is endowed with the capacity to activate a large number of exogenous chemicals, metabolically, to reactive electrophillic species, that can covalently interact with cellular DNA and other macromolecules (Miller, 1978). It is the potential alteration of the hepatocellular genome by mutational events, that forms the theoretical basis for the heritable nature of cancer as well as, at least in part, the altered phenotype of neoplastic cells (Beer and Pitot, 1989). Till now, our understanding of the exact nature of these heritable genetic alterations remains quite fragmentary.

Owing to its susceptibility to cancer induction, under a variety of conditions and because of a large body of evidence concerning the cellular, molecular biology and pathology, the liver has been examined many times, with many carcinogens for biochemical, physiological, and morphological alterations as a function of time during the development of cancer. Such studies have consistently found many cellular and tissue changes involving hepatocytes and other types of cells in the liver before the development of unequivocal hepatocellular carcinomas, the commonest form of liver cancer (Farber, 1976a). Islands of foci of hepatocytes, areas of focal hyperplasia of hepatocytes, variously designated as adenomas, regenerative nodules (Farber, 1976b) or neoplastic nodules (Squire and Levitt, 1975), hyper basophillic foci (Daoust, 1963) and generalized ductular proliferation (oval cell proliferation) in various combinations are regularly seen at different times during the carcinogenic process (Farber, 1976a; Sell, 1990).

Several studies concerned with these observations during liver carcinogenesis have been useful, indicating the cellular and tissue changes, that might be involved in a sequence important to cancer development. Nearly all such studies have involved either continuous or intermittent exposure to a carcinogen for weeks or months. Under such conditions an increasing number of overlapping sequences of events, take place, producing a wide spectrum of changes, including presumptive steps in carcinogensis, appearing simultaneously at any one moment at a time. Also discrimination between these changes are most likely to be related to cancer development and the many that are unrelated is practically impossible with such model systems.

The liver develops reversible and irreversible focal changes, and focal alterations have more than one available option. Keeping this in view, it is necessary that any model for sequential analysis of hepatocarcinogenesis, should have a limited time exposure, to each of the various stimuli or environment, so that they can exert a major modulating influence/effect on the carcinogenic process (Farber, 1980; Farber and Cameron, 1980).

5.1 Hepatocarcinogens – Classification

Chemicals known to induce liver cancer abounds in the environment, and have been classed into 5 major groups (Preusmann, 1978).

Naturally occurring hepatocarcinogens are mostly available in the plant kingdom. Carcinogenic mycotoxins, metabolites of fungi are notable. Sterigmatocystin produced by the strains of *Aspergillus versicolor* and *A. nidulans* and *A. bipolaris* is less carcinogenic than Aflatoxin B_1 (AFB_1). It has been found active in single dose experiments in mice (Fuji *et al.*, 1976). Yellow rice toxins contain 2 hepatocarcinogenic compounds–luteoskyrin and cyclochlorotine, a chlorinecontaining cyclic pentapeptide.

Hepatocarcinogens, are often environmental pollutants. Nitrosoamines abound in nitrite/nitrate treated food products such as fish, meat etc. Nitrosoamines are a group of potent and versatile carcinogens. Diethylnitrosoamine (DENA) has been observed as a potent carcinogen in 20 different animal species (Preussmann, 1975).

Organochlorine pesticides -1.1, -bis (p-Chlorophenyl) -2, 2, 2 trichloroethane (DDT), aldrin, heptachlor have been found to be carcinogenic in several strains of mice. Vinyl chloride is known to cause angiosarcoma of liver in humans. Polychlorinated biphenyls (PCBs) are carcinogenic in mouse and rat.

Drugs also serve as hepatocarcinogens. Metronidazole–a component of flagyl, was found to be carcinogenic in laboratory animals. Sex hormones such as ethinyl, oestradiol and northisterone produced liver tumours in rats.

Dyes and food colourants have strong potential to induce liver cancer in rats and mice.

Industrial chemicals such as dioxane, amitrole, trichloroethylene act as potential hepatocarcinogens.

The classification of different types of hepatocarcinogens is given in the Table 1.10.

5.2 Initiation of Liver Carcinogenesis
A Sequential Analysis

Carcinogenesis is a process, in which summation of events is required to produce a cancer. Initiation is defined as the consequences of the initial interaction of a tissue with carcinogens. While pathological changes may not be applicable, the tissue is irreversibly altered and contains cells (initiated cells) which are precusor to the future tumour.

Table 1.10 : Classification of Hepatocarcinogens

Class	*Species*	*Route*	*Source of human exposure*
A : Naturally occurring liver carcinogens	Rat, monkey duck, man	P.O	Through food.
(i) Aflatoxin B_1+ other aflatoxins			
(ii) Cycasin	Rat, mouse, hamster	P.O	Through food.
(iii) Coumarin	Rat	P.O	Through food.
B : Environmental pollutants as liver carcinogens			
(i) N-nitrosocompounds	affects		Food, respiration
DENA, DMN etc	20 species	P.O. and other routes	Cosmetics, formation in GI. tract from precursors
(ii) Vinyl chloride	mouse, rat	inhalation	Food, respiration
(iii) P.C.B.'s	Rat	P.O	Food
C : Drugs as liver carcinogens			
(i) Phenobarbital	Rat, mouse	P.O	Drug used in epilepsy, hypnotic agent.
(ii) Oxazepam	Mouse	P.O	Drug to treat psychic stress and epilepsy
(iii) Norethisterone	Mouse, rat	P.O	Drug used as oral contraceptive
D : Dyes as liver carcinogens			
(i) Auramine	Rat	P.O	Food dye
(ii) P-dimethylamino benzene (butter yellow)	Mouse, rat	P.O	Food colourant
E : Industrial chemicals as liver carcinogens			
(i) Dioxane	Rat, guineapig	P.O	Solvent
(ii) Amitrole	Mouse, rat	P.O	Herbicide

Scherer *et al.*, 1972 used either islands of altered hepatocytes or else foci of resistant hepatocytes as indices of initiation. This appears to be the first step in carcinogenesis, which is a 2-step process involving (a) induction of a biochemical event (b) fixation of some such change by a round of cell proliferation.

In the case of Scherer Emmelot model (1977), Farber's model (1978; 1979) cell proliferation in order to be effective, must occur within a few hours after carcinogen administration. This has been proved for DENA, DMH, DMN, benzo (a) pyrene (BP) and N-methyl nitroso urea (MNU).

The liver is most sensitive to initiation if a direct acting carcinogen MNU is administered between 18 and 24 hours after partial hepatectomy (Cayama *et al.,* 1978). In case of indirectly acting carcinogens such as DMH, the period of maximum susceptibility is 6 to 18 hours (Tsuda and Farber, 1979).

Thus cell injury is of considerable importance in the development of liver cancer. DNA synthesis is a major component of cell proliferation. Replication of carcinogen damaged DNA before repair (i.e. within 24 hours) or post-replication-repair (recombination) is probably of crucial importance in this process.

5.3 *Initiated Cells – Phenotypic Characteristics*

The basic nature of the alteration in cells, induced by an active carcinogen that favours or allows them to evolve into neoplasia is unknown for any system. There is no convincing evidence, in any system that such altered cells can express any degree of autonomy or growth independence even in tissues such as skin, that are programmed for continual cell proliferation (Farber and Cameron, 1980).

In the liver, available evidence does not favour the view that hepatocytes after initiation, acquired any degree of freedom for growth (Laishes and Farber, 1978). Islands of altered histochemistry induced by pH and DENA displays some inherent proliferative capacity, independent of the cytotoxic environment created by the carcinogen (Scherer and Emmelot, 1976).

The known biochemical markers for islands or foci of putative preneoplastic lesions (hepatocytes) are listed (Farber, 1980). This list is composite and does not imply that every presumed preneoplastic lesion shows all the markers. In fact the evidence already suggests that quantitative differences, if not qualitative ones exist between islands and foci and nodules. DENA–induced hepatic foci and nodules showed a different spectrum of biochemical and histochemical changes, as reported by several workers. (Pitot *et al.*, 1978; Ogawa *et al.*, 1980; Dragan *et al.*, 1994 a, b).

Foci and persistent nodules are 90% to 95% positive for GGT and 80-85% of these lesions show deficiencies of ATP-ase and G-6-pases. By contrast the number of islands that are positive for GGT is less than 50% and those deficient in ATP-ase, less than 40% (Pitot *et al.*, 1978; Scherer *et al.*, 1972) reports a much higher incidence of ATP ase plus G-6-pase in their studies.

However none of these markers is completely reliable and none is basic to the development of cancer, since more advanced lesions, especially cancers, show even greater individual variability (Pitot *et al.*, 1978a; Ogawa *et al.*, 1980).

One important property of initiated cells, is their irreversability. In the Scherer-Emmelot model, islands persist for at least 200 days in the absence of any known added environmental influence (Scherer and Emmelot, 1976). A similar persistance was observed in the model of Pitot (1978) and the Solt-Farber model using DENA (Solt and Farber, 1977). After initiation is fixed by the 2-step process, the cells persist for many months and appear not to be recognized by the host in a manner, that results in their destruction.

5.4 *Assays for Initiation*

Initiation of hepatocarcinogenesis is assayed by 3 methods:

A: Measurement of the number of islands of hepatocytes, that shows distinctive patterns of altered histochemical reactions (Pitot *et al.*, 1978; Sirica *et al.*, 1978).

B: Resistant hepatocytes that appear when the liver is subjected to can intense selection pressure for resistant cells (Solt and Farber, 1976; Tsuda and Farber, 1979; Tatematsu *et al.*, 1979).

C: Appearance of Cancer.

A and B are relatively short, lasting 4-6 weeks while C is long and may take 9 months to 2 years. A and B measure initiation while C measures not only initiation but also promotion, and the steps beyond that, involving the development of neoplasia from an early neoplastic step. The principal biochemical and enzymatic markers for preneoplastic hepatocytes are tabled (Table 1.11).

5.5 *Promotion of Initiated Hepatocytes*

Promotions, the second stage, is confined to those processes which facilitate the expression of initiated phenotype at the tissue level. Promotion may result from influence of promoting agent on the entire tissue or on the initiated cells (Yuspa and Poirier, 1988). In liver, promotion is best observed in RH model. It leads to production of focal areas of hyperplasia or regenerative nodules or neoplastic nodules. In a solid organ the liver, with highly organized architecture (Farber, 1980) focal proliferation or hyperplasia of hepatocytes could be the result of 1) Differential inhibition 2) Differential stimulation 3) Differential recovery stimulation.

Assays for Promotion

Promotion is assayed by 2 methods. A : Induction of cancer. B : Rate of induction and number of hyperplastic nodules.

Table 1.11 : Biochemical and Enzymatic Markers for Pre-neoplastic Hepatocytes

I. Negative loss of

(a) Carbohydrate metabolising enzymes eg. gluco kinase, aldolase B, pyruvate kinase I, glucose-6-phosphatase and other glyconeogenic enzymes, glycogen phosphorylase.

(b) Aminoacid metabolising enzymes. Eg. Tryptophan 2,3-dioxygenase, serine dehydratase.

(c) Drug metabolising enzymes (in Phase I) eg : cytochrome P-450's, mixed function oxygenases, arylhydrocarbon hydroxylase, glutathione peroxidase (Se-dependent).

(d) Other enzymes eg : ATPase (Ca^{++}, Mg^{++} dependent), loss of concentration ability for Iron.

II. Positive gain of

(a) Carbohydrate metabolising enzmes of glucose-6-phosphate dehydrogenase, non hepatic (foetal type) isoenzymes of glycolysis.

(b) Drug metabolising enzymes.
UDPGT-(Type I or foetal type)
Epoxide hydrolase etc.

(c) Glutathione related enzymes.
GST, GGT, GPx (Se-independent)

(d) Other enzymes.
α-Fetoprotein, preneoplastic antigen, amyl esterase etc.

A : This assay is a long term assay, requiring upto 9 months for completion (Pitot *et al.*, 1978a).

B : It is much shorter requiring 2-4 weeks (Tsuda and Farber, 1979).

5.6 *Progression*

Distinct from tumour promotion is the process of tumour progression. The changes in this stage of carcinogensis include further phenotypic alterations in the initiated cell population, indicating conversion from pre-malignant to malignant type.

5.7 *Liver Tumours – A Pathological Profile*

Sasaki and Yoshida (1935) detailed the step by step changes of liver parenchyma leading to the development of malignant liver tumours, in experimental hepatocarcinogenesis. They described the sequential appearance of foci of hyperplasia, nodular adenomas and finally hepatomas. Essential features of this process was confirmed by subsequent studies (Williams, 1980a).

5.8 *Hepatocellular Lesions*

Altered foci and neoplastic nodules are two types of hepato cellular lesions (Keysser *et al.*, 1980). Altered foci are small lesions of hepatocytes that do not disturb the parenchymal architecture. They are equivalant to hyperplastic foci (Newberne and Wogan, 1968). Neoplastic nodules are longer lesions that disrupt and compress the surrounding parenchyma. They correspond to lesions described as adenomas (Sasaki and Yoshida, 1935).

5.9 *Altered Foci*

A lesion smaller than the size of a lobule is the focus, while a lesion longer than a lobule is referred to as an "area" (Keysser, 1980). Current evidence indicates that areas are simply large foci. 2FAA produces four distinctive types of fociclear cell foci, eosinophillic or ground glass foci, basophillic foci and mixed cell foci (Squire and Levitt, 1975). Cells in eosinophillic foci are enlarged due to an increase in cytoplasm. Cells in basophillic foci have diffuse cytoplasmic basophillia and are either longer or smaller than normal hepatocytes. Clear cells are somewhat larger. Basophillic foci are more significant with respect to tumour development than other cellular alterations (Marsman and Popp, 1994). Cells in the foci have increased mitotic index. Williams *et al.* (1976) proving that lesions develop by proliferation. Foci are counted per unit area in standard sections from all lobes of the liver.

5.10 Neoplastic Nodules

Neoplastic nodules are spherical lesions that occupy an area equivalent in size to that of several liver lobules (Squire and Levitt, 1975). They appear elevated above the liver surface. Nodules exhibit compression of surrounding liver tissue. Nodules are greyish white in colour and are sharply demarcated from the surrounding reddish brown non-nodular parenchyma. Nodules lack the normal pattern of reticulum that lines the sinusoids (Williams and Watanabe, 1978). Nodular cells are of variable size and their cytoplasm stains predominently acidophillic or basophillic. Their nuclei may be enlarged and hyperchromatic. Nodules appear only after development of foci (Williams *et al.*, 1976). Nodules reveal elevated mitotic index (Williams *et al.*, 1976) and display increased DNA synthesis. Therefore it appears that nodules arise by progressive growth of foci.

In a sequential study of nodule development, all nodules persisted after removal of the carcinogen and continued to increase in size (Hirota and Williams, 1979). Thus nodules are progressively growing lesions and must be considered to be neoplastic. Nodules exhibit extensive cystic change, indicating degenerative or regressive alteration (Williams, 1980).

5.11 Hepato Cellular Carcinoma (HCC)

Several oncologists have extensively described the histopathologic characterstics of hepatocellular carcinomas (Firminger *et al.*, 1952; Williams, 1980). Carcinomas differ from neoplastic nodules, both cytologically and morphologically, as well as in the patterns of architectural arrangements. Their nuclei are a typical, showing nuclear hyperchromasia. 3 types of HCCs are recognized – trabecular, adenocarcinoma, hepato blastomas (Turusov *et al.*, 1973). HCCs display many of the functional abnormalities described for altered foci and neoplastic nodules. They are resistant to iron accumulation (Williams Yamamoto, 1972) and are characterized by a number of enzyme abnormalities (Fiala and Fiala, 1973).

The development of hepatic carcinomas is commonly preceded by numerous cellular foci which demonstrate aberrant expression of common hepatic enzymatic markers (Pitot *et al.*, 1978). A fraction of these progress to pre-malignant hepatic nodules of which a few convert to cancer (Goldfarb and Pugh 1982; Periano *et al.*, 1983).

5.12 The Growing Need for Studying Liver Tumours

On a global basis, cancer of the liver is on the rise, and is assuming alarming, dimensions. The atlas of Cancer mortality in U.S.A. reveals a high incidence of Cancer of bilary passages and liver in areas where industrial power plants-petrochemical plants are concentrated (Mason *et al.*, 1976). Areas of high incidence are Sub-Saharan Africa, South East Asia, Taiwan and main land China. In these areas there appears to be a 5:1 predominance of males to females with regard to H.C.C. In addition P.L.C. (Primary Liver Cancer) is on the rise in Latin America, and Africa. The epidemiology of liver tumours with gross variations in geographic distribution, prompts man to search for etiological factors. The liver had also been the principal focus of attention, as a target for chemical carcinogenesis, ever since Sasaki and Yoshida (1935) discovered liver cancer induction with butter yellow.

Industrial effluents as causative factors for liver cancer deserves special mention. Their carcinogenic effect is easily substantiated by epidemiological observations, because they cause lesions, otherwise rare in man. The prevalence of such tumours in a limited population, exposed to such effluents is suggestive of some sort of a causal connection between the two.

Throtust used in X-ray photography and vinyl chloride induce hepatic angio sarcoma in humans. Inhalation of vinyl chloride by rodents, produces hepatic angiosarcoma, similar to tumour appearing after vinyl chloride exposure in human populations (Popper *et al.*, 1977). This is the first prediction of human hepatocarcinogenesis from animal studies.

Finally the importance of liver tumours lies in their role in actions of regulatory agencies in evaluating carcinogenic agents. Hepatic tumours are the principal parameters in these decisions since it is presumed that an agent carcinogenic for the liver may reflect carcinogenicity for other organs.

For practical reasons, experiments on carcinogenesis are carried out on rodents. Species differences in microsomal biotransformation systems, both with regard to the formation and degradation of active metabolites, may account for their increased tendency to tumour formation.

What remains the most baffling problem is the extrapolation of animal data to man. Not only do the experimental animals live under well defined control conditions, free of exercise and often of sex, but even more important is the great genetic heterogeneity of man, in contrast to experimental animals.

Popper (1978) has stated that a small fraction of human population exposed to a strong carcinogen have cancer. But even if only a small percentage of man exposed to carcinogen develop carcinoma, the total number in the human population becomes exorbitant. The assessment of the balance between risk and benefit is in principle not scientific but a political decision. Explanation of pathogenesis may provide the only reliable answer that science can offer (Table 1.12).

6. Cancer Chemo Prevention

Identifying the most effective cancer-preventive agents from a pool of hundreds of promising compounds, requires a strategic approach, that includes defined criteria and decision points, based on efficacy and safety data (Greenwald *et al.*, 1993). NCI's chemopreventive agent development programme includes preclinical *in vitro* and *in vivo* screening and when warranted, human clinical trial (Malone *et al.*, 1989).

Toxicologic and safety evaluation in animals, measure the acute, subchronic, and chronic effects of the proposed chemopreventive agents. This step includes carcinogenesis studies as well as multigeneration reproductive teratogenicity studies. Compounds that exhibit high efficacy and low toxicity in these pre-clinical tests are considered for preliminary evaluation in human phase I and II clinical trials in usually limited number of high risk, but otherwise healthy subjects.

Table 1.12 : DENA - The Better Choice as Experimental Hepatocarcinogen

- It has low hepatotoxic but high hepatocarcinogenic properties.
- It has been observed to be carcinogenic in about 20 different types of laboratory animals.
- DENA produces liver cancer in rats slowly, following a single oral, intravenous or intraperitoneal administration.
- It can be produced *in vivo* from injested secondary amines and nitrate compounds.
- It is found in different food products.
- It is a component of cosmetics, petrol and lubricant additives.

6.1 *In Vitro Testing*

The preclinical evaluation of potential chemopreventive agents, begins with a series of *in vitro* screening tests. *In vitro* systems provide a method for rapidly selecting and prioritizing promising agents for *in vivo* testing. *In vitro* assays evaluate the potential cancer preventive activity of new agents, using cell transformation systems. The battery of assays can be used to predict whether the agents being tested, possess anti-initiator and/ or antipromoter activity (Greenwald *et al.*, 1991). The strengths of an *in vitro* testing are A : efficiency in terms of cost and time in the evaluation of a given agent.

B : Sensitivity and ease of quantification.

C : Controlled test conditions.

D : Potential use of human cells.

Both cell and tissue systems, cultured with specific carcinogens are employed and includes as well, systems derived from human material. This helps provide a species-specific screen not suitable in animal models.

6.2 *In Vivo Testing*

Agents demonstrating clear efficacy in the *in vitro* screens, are evaluated further, using a battery of *in vivo* efficacy and safety tests.

In vivo screening provides, the initial evidence of positive chemopreventive activity in carcinogen-induced animal tumour models, establishes an initial dose response for compound efficacy and toxicity; and provides evidence of agent acceptability and tolerance in mammals (Malone *et al.*, 1989; Boone *et al.*, 1990). Several criteria have been established to determine the battery of *in vivo* models to be used in chemoprevention agent development. Since target organ systems must be relevant to human cancers, *in vivo* animal models for lung, liver, colon, breast and skin have to be chosen. Models using multistage carcinogensis are included, as are chemical models with or without activation.

6.3 *Cancer Chemo Prevention – Objective – Basic Mechanism*

The aim of cancer chemoprevention is to circumvent the development and progression of precancerous cells through the use of non-cytotoxic nutrients and/or pharmacologic agents. Since the time span between tumour initiation and frank malignancy, often exceeds a decade, there is a considerable time frame, within which the carcinogenic process could be halted or reversed (Alberts and Garcia, 1995). Although decreasing cancer incidence and mortality are the ultimate goals of cancer chemoprevention, yet much effort is to be devoted, towards identifying specific steps in the carcinogenesis process, that are amenable to intervention and can serve as surrogate end point biomarkers for possible modulation by chemopreventive agents.

At least 2 basic mechanisms seem noteworthy, and show how chemopreventive agents with low toxicity inhibit carcinogenesis. Fig. 3 identifies the potential sites of action of inhibitors of chemical carcinogenensis. Numbers denote sites where inhibitors are effective (Slaga, 1991).

Chemopreventive agents may act by altering the manner in which the carcinogen is handled by the organism prior to the time it reacts with the critical target site(s).

Second, such agents may act later by altering the biologic properties of cells, that already have been subjected to the effects of chemical carcinogens, in the multi stage process of carcinogenesis (Table 1.13).

6.4 Chemo Preventive Agents – Classes

Table 1.13 depicts the various classes of chemopreventive agents :-

Compounds, which exert their action by inhibiting the formation of carcinogens have been studied in detail (Mirvish, 1981a, b).

-tocopherol and phenols inhibit formation of n-Nitroso compounds (Newmark and Mergens, 1981).

Blocking agents prevent carcinogens from reacting with critical target sites. Disulfuram prevents symmetrical DMH induced neoplasia of the large bowel (Wattenberg, 1975). Physiological nucleophiles such as glutathione, and xenobiotic components present in the plant constituents of the diet, scaverge the ultimate carcinogenic form of B.P. Ellagic acid is a very potent blocking agent in this regard (Wood *et al.*, 1982).

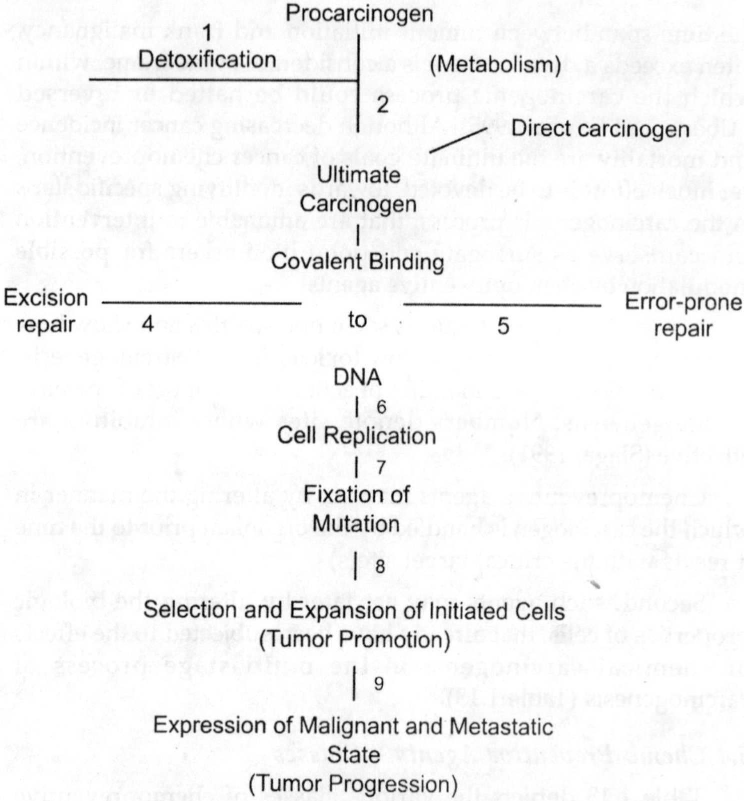

Fig. 1.3 : Potential sites of action of inhibitors of chemical carcinogenesis. Number represents sites where inhibitors may be effective (Slaga, 1991).

Suppressing agents refer to compounds that inhibit carcinogenesis, when administered subsequent to a course of carcinogen administration that would result in the formation of cancers. Beta carotene and selenium salts are suppressing agents that inhibits a considerable variety of experimental neoplastic systems (Han, 1993; Ip *et al.*, 1994; Ip and Lisk, 1994; Rana *et al.*, 1998 a, b).

In addition to these, these are also another group of inhibitors that helps prevent attack by oxygen radicals, thereby inhibiting tumour promotion (Perchellet and Perchellet, 1989). Phenolic anti oxidants inhibits tumour promotion by benzoyl peroxide and TPA (Slaga *et al.*, 1983; Agarwal *et al.*, 1992).

Table 1.13 : Chemopreventive Agents : Classes

A. Chemopreventive agents, effective against complete carcinogens:

Egs :

(a) Compounds inhibiting formation of carcinogens eg. -Tocopherol, Phenols.

(b) Blocking agents
Eg : glutathione

(c) Suppressing agent
Eg : Selenium salts, plant sterols and flavones.

B. Chemopreventive agents useful against tumour promotion

Eg : L-methionine
s - adenosyl-L-methionine.

C. Chemopreventive agents effective when administered shortly before exposure to carcinogens.

Eg : 2(3) tert-butyl-hydroxyanisole.

L-methionine, S-adenosyl L-methionine exert inhibitory influences during promotion of chemically induced rat liver carcinogenesis (Garcea, *et al.*, 1989; Pascale, *et al.*, 1991). Finally some chemopreventive agents have been found effective, when administered shortly before exposure to a carcinogen. These include Kahweol palmitate, Benzylisothiocyanate etc. (Wattenberg and Lam, 1984; Wattenberg, 1985).

7. Objectives of the Present Study

The present book is an attempt to show the anticarcinogenic potential of the medicinal plant *Trianthema portulacastrum* L in experimentally induced chemical rat hepatocarcinogenesis. The objective of the work incorporated in this book is an outcome of the lacunae in the existing scientific knowledge, regarding the tremendous possibility of herbal medicine in curing the dreaded killer disease. In this book a careful attempt has been made to evaluate the role of *Trianthema portulacastrum* in experimental hepatocarcinogeneis.

Briefly the objectives are as follows:

- To ascertain whether *Trianthema portularcastrum* L has anticarcinogenic potential against experimentally induced hepatocarcinogenesis.
- If functional to determine the optimum dose for regression of neoplasia, devoid of toxic manifestation.

- To identify the fraction/fractions exhibiting maximum anti-hepatocarcinogenic activity.
- To characterize the stage(s) in the carcinogenic process, where the plant extract is most effective in the reversion of preneoplastic pathology, thus delaying neoplasia.
- To correlate various biological and biochemical events to arrive at a meaningful explanation of the chemopreventive role of the extract in experimental hepatocarcinogenesis.
- To focus on the unknown mechanism of action of the plant extract at the cellular, sub-cellular, chromosomal level. The experimental regimen included in the book reflects the above objectives.

2

Anti-Carcinogenic Potential of Different Fractions of *Trianthema portulacastrum* L.

A Morphometric Analysis in One-stage and Two-stage Rat Hepatocarcinogenesis

1. Introduction

Hepatocarcinogenesis in rats can be induced by various carcinogens such as 2-acetylaminofluorene (2-AAF), Diethylnitrosoamine (DENA). Dimethylnitrosoamine (DMNA), P-dimethylaminoazobenzene (P-DAB), Aflatoxin B_1 (AFB_1). It is a multistep process (Farber, 1980). Several models of rat hepatocarcinogenesis have evolved, to examine the competence of various compounds, to modulate the carcinogenic process. (Moreno *et al.*, 1991; Tsuda *et al.*, 1994). In most models, focal areas of altered hepatocytes, become grossly visible nodules (hyperplastic nodules) and precede the appearance of malignant tumours (Kaneko *et al.*, 1980; Scherer *et al.*, 1984; Farber, *et al.*, 1976c). The histochemical and ultra structural features of hepatocytes, constituting the nodules, are different from those of normal adult rat liver cells (Farber, 1973; Farber, 1977). Preneoplastic lesions can be easily identified, counted and their number and size determined by quantitative morphometry to measure multi stage hepatic carcinogenesis and its alteration by Chemo preventive agents (Moreno *et al.*, 1991).

In this study, the inhibitory effect of the different fractions of the plant extract in chemically induced rat hepatocarcinogenesis was investigated by morphometric evaluation of pre-neoplastic lesions and assessment of hepatic histopathology during the early stages of neoplastic transformation, in order to enlighten us about the potential of the extract(s) as a chemopreventive agent.

2. Materials and Methods

2.1 Plant Material

Dried overground parts of the plant *T. portulacastrum* L. were supplied by United Chemical and Allied Products, Calcutta, India. The plant was authenticated by the Botanical Survey of India and a voucher specimen no: (Ju/Pharm/Biochem/SP03), has been deposited in the same herbarium.

2.2 Extraction of Plant Material

Air dried, overground plants of *T. portulacastrum* L. were crushed in a waring blender and the fine pulverized material was subjected to exhaustive extraction in a Soxhlet's extractor, with petroleum ether (b.p 60-80°C). The pet-ether extract was discarded. The marc was then successively extracted with benzene, choloroform, acetone and finally ethanol 95% w/v (Vohra and Shah, 1983). The liquid concentrate obtained in case of the chloroform extract and ethanolic extract were separately subjected to distillation, in a distillating flask, using a glass condenser. Each distillation took about 60 minutes. The extract in each case was taken in a round bottomed flask, placed within a heating mantle. The distillate was collected in another flat bottomed flask. The flask containing the extract and the flask containing the final distilled product, were connected to a condenser, connected to a water source by rubber tubing. The heating mantle was inturn fitted to an electric source. The distillate observed in each case, were eventually reduced to solid residues by rotary vacuum evaporation below 45°C to yield 4.6% w/w and 4.8% w/w of chloroform and alcohol fractions respectively. These were stored at 4°C until used.

The chloroform fraction and the ethanolic fractions were separately suspended in deionized water prior to anticarcinogenic evaluation 0.2 ml of 0.05% Tween 80 was added to the sticky chloroform fraction in distilled water using a Potter-Elvehjhum homogeniser. Tween 80 was added as an emulsifying agent to enhance the solubility of the fraction in water. Crude aqueous extract of *T. portulacastrum* was prepared by refluxing in double distilled water and concentrated under vacuum. (Speed Vac Sc 110 A, Virginia, U.S.A.) (Devi and Ganasoundari, 1995).

2.3 Animals and Diet

Male sprague dawley rats were obtained from Indian Institute of Chemical Biology (C.S.I.R.), Calcutta. The animals weighed 100-120 g at the time of initial purchase. All rats were maintained on semi-purified basal diet and water adlibitum, until the body weights reached 130-150 g range. The composition of the semipurified basal diet is stated in Table 2.1 (Aquino *et al.*, 1985). The diet is well balanced and includes vitamins, minerals, aminoacids for normal healthy up-keep of laboratory animals. (Table 2.1).

2.4 Experimental Regimen : One Stage Hepatocarcinogenesis

Rats were divided at random into experimental and control groups with 10-12 rats per group. Group A' animals were *Trianthema* controls and received crude *Trianthema* extract and Tween 80. Group A animal constituted the normal untreated controls and received no DENA treatment. Initiation of hepatocarcinogenesis was performed by a single intraperitoneal injection of Diethylnitrosoamine (DENA), Sigma chemical Co : St. Louis, M.O, U.S.A. at a dose of 200 mgs/kg body weight in 0.9% NaCl solution. Stewart *et al.*, 1980; Pitot *et al.*, 1978a; i.p injection of DENA was administered to all the groups B, C, D and E. Group B animals were the carcinogen controls. They received only DENA and no other treatment. Group C animals received DENA and were administered crude aqueous extract of *T. portulacastrum* at the dose of 100 mgs/kg body weight per animal once daily from the day of carcinogen administration throughout the course of study. Group D animals received DENA and were administered ethanolic extract of *T. portulacastrum* at the dose of 100 mgs/kg body weight per animal once daily concomittant with DENA administration, till the end of the study.

Group E animals also received DENA and were treated with 100 mgs/kg body weight of chloroform extract of *T. portulacastrum*, to the basal diet, of each animal once daily till the end of the experiment. Group A' animals (*Trianthema* controls) received the plant drug at the same dose. EtOH control and chloroform control animals (data not shown) also received the extract in Tween 80 i.e. 100 mgs/kg body weight/animal once daily throughout the course of the study.

Table 2.1 : Composition of the Semi-purified Basal Diet

Components (Candida utilis)	*Amount of the substance present by weight*
Torula yeast	40.0
Sucrose	37.9
Dextrin	10.0
Cellulose	4.0
Corn-oil	5.0
D-L-methionine	0.5
Mineral mix a	2.1
Vitamin mix b	0.5

a = (provided in gm/kg diet);

$CaCO_3$ 19.6; NaCl 1.2; $MnSO_4$ 0.06 and KI 0.001.

b = { (Provided per kg diet) retinyl acetate 1,250 I.u, cholecalciferol 120 I.u; menadione 100 g; vitamin B12 (Cyanocobalamin 5 g and Tocopheryl acetate 200 mgs).

After 22 weeks on this regimen, animals were sacrificed, and morphometric evaluations made.

2.5 *Morphology and Morphometry*

After exactly 22 weeks on the regimen, animals were weighed, and then the rats were sacrificed under light ether anaesthesia, and fasted overnight prior to sacrifice. After sacrifice, livers were excised, blotted dry, quickly weighed (Table 2.2) and examined on the surface for visible macroscopic liver lesions-neoplastic nodules. The greyish white liver lesions were easily recognized and distinguished from the surrounding non-nodular reddish brown liver parenchyma. The nodules were spherical in shape and were measured in two perpendicular directions, to the nearest millimetre, to obtain the average diameter of each nodule. Nodules were divided into 3 categories, in accordance with their respective size, total area of liver parenchyma occupied – (≤ 1 m), > 1-<3 mm and ≥ 3 mm) as described by Moreno *et al.*, (Moreno *et al.*, 1991; Bishayee *et al.*, 1995). The nodule incidence percentage, total number of nodules, and nodule multiplicity were calculated (Table 2.3). From the measured diameters, individual nodule volume and nodule volume as percentage of total liver volume were calculated (Table 2.4).

For histological preparations, representative slices, were excised from right, left and caudate lobes of each liver, quickly fixed in 10% neutral buffered formalin. At least two slices per liver were embedded in paraffin and were microtomed (5 μm thick) and stained with haematoxylin and Eosin. Histological slides were scanned in different planes under a photomicrocope for specific hepatocellular lesions. Altered hepatocyte foci were counted (No:/cm^2) and their number and size were calculated according to published criteria (Bannasch, 1976; Stewart *et al.*, 1980, Moreno *et al.*, 1991). The exact percentage of liver parenchyma occupied by focal lesions was also taken into consideration (Table 2.5) (Moreno *et al.*, 1991).

2.6 *Statistical Analysis*

The statistical analysis for hepatocellular lesions in different groups was performed by Fisher's exact probability test. All other data were analysed by students t-test.

3. Results

3.1 *Food and Water Intakes*

There was no observable treatment related change, in the average daily food and water intake among the different experimental animals.

Mortality

All animals survived, during the entire course, of the experiment.

3.2 *Body and Liver Weights of Rats During the Period of Experiment*

Table 2.2 depicts the final body weights of the animals in grams, liver weight also in grams and the relative liver weights, in the experimental animals, sacrificed on the 22nd week following DENA administration. There was a slight decrease, in the final body weight of rats, subjected to DENA (carcinogen) alone i.e. Group B in comparison to Group A (i.e. normal untreated controls). The result is statistically significant. In the groups C, D and E undergoing treatment with different fractions of *T. portulacastrum*, animals maintained near normal body weights, indicating clearly that the crude aqueous, EtOH and $CHCl_3$ fractions had no toxic effect on the growth responses of the rats, and was fairly well tolerated. The relative liver weights did not vary significantly betwen the groups. In Group E and in Group C, the variation was significant, $P<0.05$ compared is Group B (DENA Control) group by student's t-test. In Group B the change in liver weight was significant $P<0.02$ as compared to Group A (Table 2.2). Control animals displayed bodyweight, liver weight, relative liver weight close to the normal untreated group (Group A).

3.3 Hepatic Neoplastic Nodules

Administration of the aqueous, EtOH and $CHCl_3$ extracts of the medicinal plant *Trianthema portulacastrum* L. at a dose of 100 mgs/kg body weight, to the basal diet of each animal once daily, brought about a significant reduction of nodule incidence in DENA induced rat hepatocarcinogenesis (Table 2.3). In the DENA control group, receiving the carcinogen alone, the nodule incidence was 100%. It dropped to 54.5% in the EtOH fraction, 50% in the aqueous fraction treated groups and was remarkably low in Group E (i.e. chloroform–extract treated group). In this group nodule incidence was only 25%. In groups C and E $P < 0.01$ compared to DENA-control group by Fisher's exact probability test and in Group D $P < 0.02$ compared to the DENA control group by Fisher's exact probability test.

The average number of nodules, per nodule bearing animal (nodule multiplicity) were also considered in the study. In Group D $P < 0.02$, in Group C $P < 0.01$ and in Group E, $P < 0.001$ compared to DENA control group by student's t-test.

Table 2.4 depicts the size distribution and growth of DENA induced hepatic nodules, in the different groups of rats. Mean nodular volume and nodule volume, as percentage of liver volume is shown after 22 weeks of plant drug supplementation. A notable observation in the study, was the reduction in the appearance of nodules greater than 3 mm in all the extract treated groups (i.e. Groups C,D,E), compared to the carcinogen control group (i.e. Group B). Mean nodular volume showed a decrease from 1.61 cm^3 in Group B to 0.93 cm^3 in Group D, 0.81 cm^3 in Group C and 0.75 cm^3 in group E. The aqueous, EtOH and most remarkably the $CHCl_3$ fraction treated groups, revealed a reduced nodular volume/liver volume percent. In the groups C and D, $P < 0.05$ compared to DENA control group by student's t-test and in Group E, $P < 0.001$ compared to DENA control group by student's t-test. The results are statistically significant.

3.4 Altered Hepatocyte Foci

The effect of the different extracts of *Trianthema portulacastrum* on the growth and development of altered hepatocyte foci, induced by DENA in rats is given in Table 2.5. There was a remarkable decrease in the incidence of altered foci expressed in terms of percentage from 100% in carcinogen control group (Group B) to 72.7% in Group C, to 75% in Group D and 58.33% in Group E. The percentage area of liver parenchyma, occupied by foci was significantly reduced in all the plant extract treated groups i.e. Groups C, D, E. There was also a reduction in the number of foci/cm^2 in the extract treated groups. $P < 0.05$ in groups C and D compared to Group B.

In Group D, $P < 0.02$, in Group C, $P < 0.01$ and in Group E $P < 0.01$ compared to DENA control group by Fisher's exact probability test.

3.5 Histologic Profile of Rat Liver in DENA–Induced Hepato Carcinogenesis

In Group A, livers displayed normal hepatocellular architecture, with no signs of any apparent abnormality. In Group B, numerous hepatocellular lesions, were apparent. The lesions were altered hepatocyte foci and nodules, dispersed throughout the liver parenchyma. In H & E stained hepatic sections, focal changes were demarcated from surrounding normal parenchyma. Altered hepatocytes of foci were of four principal types–clear cell, eosinophillic, basophillic and mixed cell types. Group B animals, showed numerical preponderance of eosinophillic foci rather than mixed or clear cell foci after 22 weeks of study. In Groups C, D, E clear cell foci by contrast to eosinophillic or mixed cell foci, were found to predominate. In Group E, animals treated with chloroform extract of *Trianthema portulacastrum,* the liver cells, showed nearly normal hepatocellular architecture comparable to Group A animals (normal controls).

4. Discussion

The morphometric study clearly demonstrates that the plant *Trianthema portulacastrum* L is a very promising plant, so long as the anticarcinogenic property is concerned. The present investigation, demonstrated that the chloroform extract of *T. portulacastrum* L along with other fractions, could bring about marked reduction of DENA induced rat hepatocarcinogenesis at least at the dose under observation. The chloroform extract was remarkable, in that it was able to suppress nodule development/hepatocellular lesion formation in rats, to such a degree, that in most rats of Group E, nodule development was practically nil, or if nodules developed, it was very feeble and very much reduced in size (Figs. 1 and 2).

From the study it is clearly visualized that following treatment with *T. portulacastrum* extracts, particularly the chloroform extract, in DENA injected animals, lesser number of rats developed nodules and revealed a smaller average number of nodules/nodule bearing liver, than in the group in which the carcinogen was administered alone. Plant drug contained in the fractions of *T. portulacastrum* L. also inhibited to a great extent, the appearanceof nodules >3 mm in size with subsequent reduction of nodular volume and also reduction in the nodular volume as a percentage of liver volume.

The body weights of the experimental animals, may be considered to be more or less uniform. The lowering of nodule incidence appears to be unconnected with the nutritional status of the experimental animals. Animals took the normal food and water intakes and the plant extracts, did not affect this intake of food and water, indicating that the plant extract was apparently non-toxic and therefore well tolerated by the animals. This is to be given due cognizance as nutritional deprivation causing body weight loss, may parallel a decrease in tumour volume (Waitzberg *et al.*, 1989). Further the extract could confer a great degree of protection against chemical hepatocarcinogenesis, particularly that initiated by DENA. There is, however, ample evidence to indicate that hepatic preneoplastic lesions are putative precursors of hepatocellular carcinoma in rats and perhaps also in human

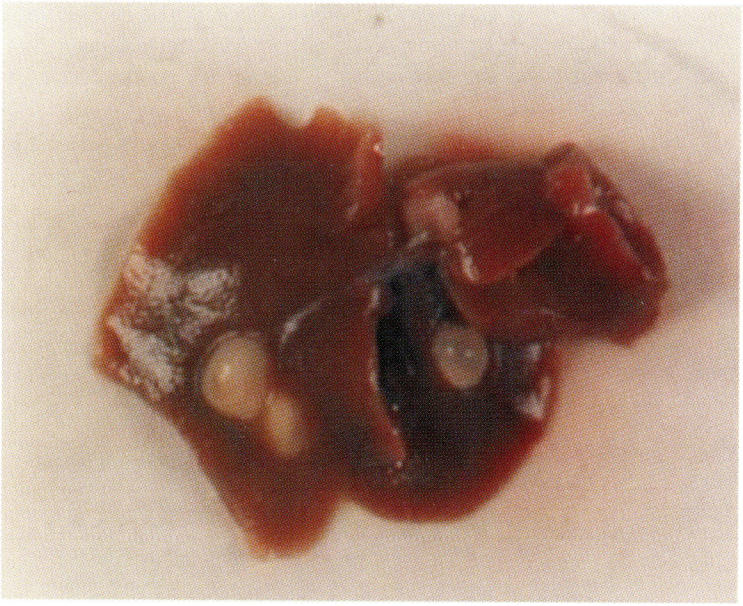

Fig. 1 : DENA treated liver showing nodules.

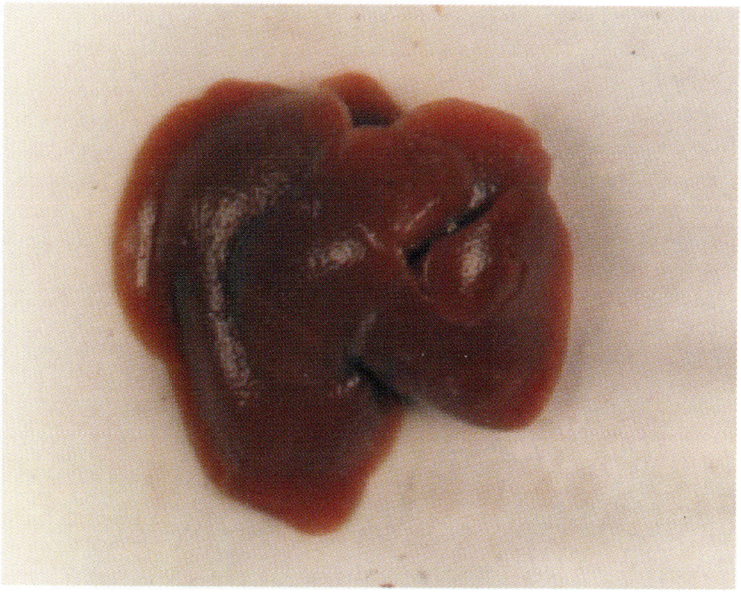

Fig. 2 : Liver returning to normalcy after drug administration. ($CHCl_3$ extract of *T. portulacastrum* L.)

beings (Scherer and Emmelot, 1975a,b; Pitot and Sirica, 1980; Williams, 1980b). The existing data suggest that liver altered foci represent neoplasia development in an experimental model system and this seems to be an important characteristic for evaluating the consistent manner in which foci appear, during post initiation events in rat hepatocarcinogenesis (Pitot *et al.*, 1980; Rabes, 1972; Farber *et al.*, 1976a).

Since there is a strong correlation between foci and hepatocarcinogenesis, our observed data, proves beyond doubt that the administration of the plant extracts can remarkably affect post-initiation stages of hepatocarcinogenesis and may perhaps affect the power with which DENA induces foci to appear (Bhattacharya *et al.*, 1998).

Table 2.2 : Body and Liver Weight of Rats Belonging to Different Experimental Groups-I Stage Morphometry

Group		*No. of rats*	*Final body weight (g)*	*Liver weight (g)*	*Relative liver weight (g liver/ 100 gm body weight)*
A'	Trianthema control	10	313.2 ± 29.1	10.4 ± 2.4	3.32 ± 0.32
A	Normal control	10	314.1 ± 24.6[a]	10.5 ± 2.2	3.34 ± 0.15
B	DENA control	10	301.2 ± 21.1	14.0 ± 3.4	4.64 ± 0.47[b]
C	Aqueous Extract of T.P + DENA	12	311.9 ± 37.0	10.1 ± 2.0	3.23 ± 0.32[c]
D	EtOH extract of T.P + DENA	11	305.1 ± 28.6	12.2 ± 2.6	3.99 ± 0.40
E	$CHCl_3$ extract of T.P + DENA	12	312.7 ± 32.8	10.3 ± 2.2	3.29 ± 0.35[c]

[a] Value represents the mean ± SE.

[b] $P < 0.02$ compared to normal control group by students t-test.

[c] $P < 0.05$ compared to DENA control group by students t-test.

Table 2.3 : Chemopreventive Efficacy of *T. portulacastrum* on the Development of DENA-Induced Hepatic Nodules.

Group		*No. of rats with nodules /total rats*	*Nodule incidence (%)*	*Total number of nodules*	*Average Number of of nodules/nodule bearing liver. (nodule multiplicity)*
A'	Trianthema control	-	-	-	-
A	Normal control	-	-	-	-
B	DENA control	10/10	100	335	33.5 ± 3.2[a]
C	Aqueous extract of T.P. + DENA	6/12	50[d]	119	19.8 ± 2.1[e]
D	EtOH extract of T.P. + DENA	6/11	54.5[b]	131	21.8 ± 2.8[c]
E	$CHCl_3$ extract of T.P. + DENA	3/12	25.0[d]	22	7.3 ± 0.9[f]

[a] Value represents the mean ± SE.

[b] P < 0.02 and [d] P < 0.01 compared to DENA control group by Fischer's exact probability test.

[c] P < 0.02, [e] P < 0.01 and [f] P < 0.001 compared to DENA control group by students t-test.

Most of the antineoplastic agents available in the market produce many toxic side effects like nephrotoxicity, cirrhosis etc. (Cleave *et al.*, 1980; Thompson *et al.*, 1984), but since the experimental animals indulged in normal food and water intakes, the extract may be taken to be non-toxic.

A fundamental question may however strike our mind– How does the plant extract exerts its influence on DENA-induced hepatocarcinogensis? It has been reported that DENA confers carcinogenic action by its metabolic conversion to a reactive ethylating agent, that can alkylate cellular DNA (Magee *et al.*, 1976; Bartsch *et al.*, 1989). The inhibitory effect of the plant extract in DENA - induced hepatocarcinogenesis is likely to be related to the detoxification of the carcinogen, through inhibition or by induction of enzymes.

Table 2.4 : Chemopreventive Role of *T. portulacastrum* on the Size Distribution and Growth of DENA-Induced Hepatic Nodules in Rats

Group	*No. of rats*	*Size of the Nodules*			*Mean nodular volume[a] (cm³)*	*Nodular volume/ liver volume[b] (%)*
		≤ 1 mm	*≥1-≤ 3 mm*	*≥ 3 mm*		
A' Trianthema control	-	-	-	-	-	-
A Normal control	-	-	-	-	-	-
B DENA control	10	85	130	120	1.61±0.27[c]	67.3±5.9
C Aqueous extract of T.P. + DENA	6	40	46	33	0.81±0.09[e]	48.7±4.5[d]
D EtOH extract of T.P. + DENA	6	39	50	42	0.93±0.14[d]	50.3±4.6[d]
E $CHCl_3$ extract of T.P. + DENA	3	11	8	3	0.75±0.06[f]	31.9±3.2[g]

[a] Individual nodule volumes were calculated from 2 perpendicular diameters measured on each nodule.

[b] 1 gm liver was assumed to occupy 1 cm³.

[c] Value represents the mean ± S.E.

[d] P<0.05, [e]P<0.02, [f]P<0.01 and [g]P<0.001 compared to DENA control group by students t-test.

Since the chloroform extract, appeared to be the most active fraction, inhibiting chemically induced rat hepatocarcinogenesis, it was decided to design a separate experimental protocol and proceed to 2-stage hepatocarcinogenesis, to identify the stage/ stages at which the extract exerts maximum activity as a potential chemopreventive agent (Tables 2.2, 2.3, 2.4, 2.5).

Table 2.5 : Effect of *T. portulacastrum* on the Development and Growth of Altered Liver Cell Foci Induced by DENA in Rats

Group	*No. of rats with foci/ total rats*	*Foci incidence (%)*	*No. of foci/cm²*	*Mean focal area (mm²)*	*% area of liver parenchyma occupied by foci*
A' Triantheme control	-	-	-	-	-
A Normal control	-	-	-	-	-
B DENA control	10/10	100	20.01±2.45[a]	0.38±0.06	2.91±0.19
C Aqueous extract of T.P. + DENA	8/11	72.7	12.71±1.85[b]	0.20±0.05[b]	2.10±0.16[b]
D EtOH extract of T.P. + DENA	9/12	75.0	13.11±1.75[b]	0.22±0.04[b]	2.25±0.13[c]
E $CHCl_3$ extract of T.P. + DENA	7/12	58.33[e]	11.15±1.52[d]	0.15±0.02[d]	1.62±0.06[f]

[a] Value represents the mean ± SE.

[b] P<0.05, [c]P<0.02, [d]P<0.01 and [f]P<0.01 compared to DENA control group by students t-test.

[e]P<0.05 compared to DENA control group by Fischer's exact probability test.

II Experimental Hepatocarcinogenesis–2 stage Model with Chloroform Extract (Active Component) of *Trianthema portulacastrum* Linn, (Aizoaceae)

1. Introduction

The identification of the three stages of chemical carcinogenesis i.e. initiation, promotion, progression, has paved the way for a new avenue of prevention of neoplastic growth. Any interference with one or more of these steps, would disrupt the entire process (Moreno *et al.*, 1991). Periano (1978) was the pioneer in introducing the chronic enzyme induction model, a model based on 2-stage concept of hepatocarcinogenesis.

In the previous 1 stage experiment, the observation that chloroform extract of *Trianthema portulacastrum* L. was extremely effective in arresting DENA induced rat hepatocarcinogenesis, without any toxic manifestation prompted, the design of a separate experimental protocol, to ascertain the stage/stages where the extract exerts maximum anti-tumorigenic response. In the previous experiment, the chemopreventive action of the extract was mediated through the inhibition of altered liver cell foci and hepatic nodule growth during preneoplasia, neoplasia formation. In this study, different fractions of *T. portulacastrum* were administered, during the entire course of the experiment, and so it was not possible to identify at which time point, the extract was most effective. The present study is designed to get an insight into the anticarcinogenic potential of the extract, before initiation as well as during early promotion phase of chemically induced rat hepatocarcinogenesis.

2. Materials and Methods

2.1 *Plant Material*

Dried overground parts of the plant *Trianthema portulacastrum* L. (Aizoaceae) were supplied by United Chemicals and Allied Products, Calcutta, India. The plant was authenticated by the Botanical Survey of India and a voucher specimen number (Ju/Pharm/Biochem/SP03) has been deposited in the same herbarium.

2.2 *Extraction of Plant Material*

The plant material was crushed in a waring blender and the fine pulverized material was subjected to extraction in a Soxhlet's extractor, with petroleum ether (b.p. 60-80°C). The petroleum ether extract was discarded. The residue was excessively extracted with benzene, chloroform acetone. The chloroform extract was taken in a conical flask, and then subjected to distillation. The concentrated distillate was subsequently evaporated in vacuo, and the material contained 4.8% w/w of the active component. The sample was stored at 4°C until use. Prior to anticarcinogenic evaluation, 0.2 ml of 0.05% Tween 80 was added to the sample and diluted with double distilled water. Tween 80 was added as an emulsifying agent to increase solubility of the extract in water. The sample was homogenized in a Potter-Elvehjhum homogeniser prior to administration.

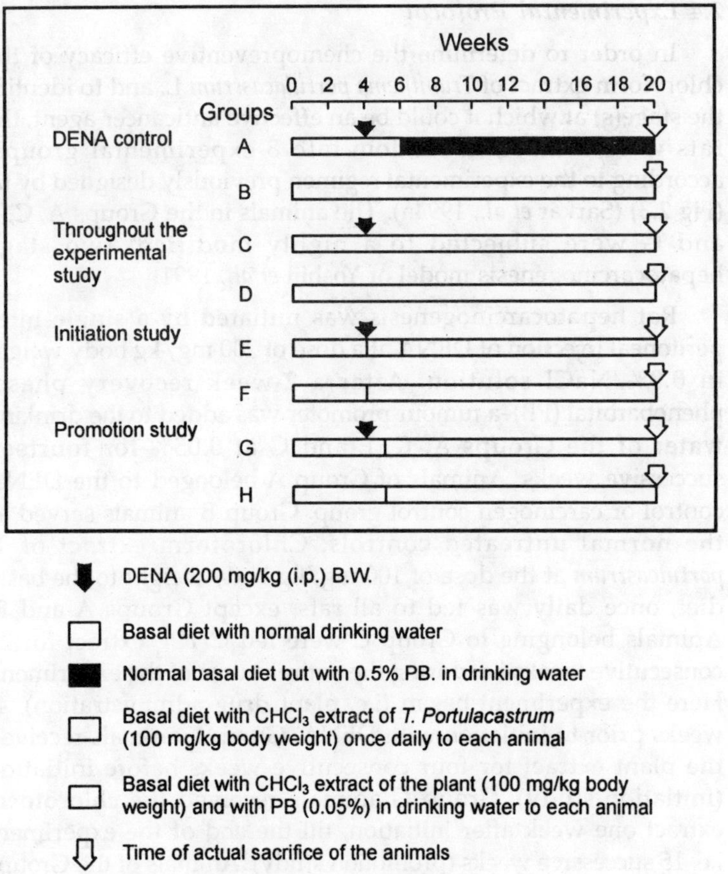

Fig. 3 : Experimental Regimen.

2.3 *Animals and Diet*

Male sprague dawley rats weighing 110-120 g were obtained from Indian Institute of Chemical Biology, C.S.I.R, Calcutta, India. These animals were used for the entire study, and were housed, 10 rats per cage in galvanized metallic cages. The animals were acclamatized to the standard laboratory conditions (temperature 25±1°C, relative humidity 60±5% and a 6 am to 6 pm photoperiod) one week prior to the actual commencement of the experiment. The animals were supplied semipurified basal diet. (Aquino *et al.*, 1985) and double distilled demineralized drinking water adlibitum.

2.4 *Experimental Protocol*

In order to determine the chemopreventive efficacy of the chloroform extract of *Trianthema portulacastrum* L. and to identify the stage(s) at which it could be an effective anticancer agent, the rats were divided at random into 8 experimental groups, according to the experimental regimen previously designed by us (Fig 2.3) (Sarkar *et al.*, 1994a). The animals in the Groups A, C, E and G were subjected to a highly modified, two stage hepatocarcinogenesis model of Yoshiji *et al.*, 1991.

Rat hepatocarcinogenesis was initiated by a single intra peritoneal injection of DENA at a dose of 200 mg/kg body weight in 0.9% NaCl solution. After a 2-week recovery phase, phenobarbital (PB)–a tumour promoter was added to the drinking water of the Groups A, C, E and G at 0.05% for fourteen successive weeks. Animals of Group A belonged to the DENA control or carcinogen control group. Group B animals served as the normal untreated controls. Chloroform extract of *T. portulcastrum* at the dose of 100 mg/kg body weight to the basal diet, once daily was fed to all rats, except Groups A and B. Animals belonging to Group C were fed $CHCl_3$ extract for 20 consecutive weeks i.e. during the entire course of the experiment. Here the experiment began (i.e. plant drug administration), 4-weeks prior to initiation with DENA. Group E animals received the plant extract for four consecutive weeks before initiation (initiation study). Group G animals received the chloroform extract one week after initiation, till the end of the experiment i.e. 15 successive weeks (promotion study). Animals of the Groups D, F and H, served as $CHCl_3$-extract controls and received in their basal diet, the extract for 20, 4 and 15 consecutive weeks. All animals were sacrificed under light ether anaesthesia, 20 weeks after the start of the experiment.

2.5 *Morphometric Evaluation in Rat Hepatocarcinogenesis–Two Stage Model*

Rats were sacrificed under light ether anaesthesia and fasted overnight prior to sacrifice. After sacrifice, livers were excised, blotted dry, weighed and examined on the surface for visible macroscopic liver lesions (neoplastic nodules). Greyish white sub-capsular nodules were easily discernable from the surrounding reddish brown, non-nodular parenchyma. The spherical nodules, were measured in two perpendicular directions, to the nearest millimetre, to obtain the average diameter of each nodule. Nodules were divided into 3 categories in accordance with their respective size, total area of liver parenchyma occupied (≤1 mm, > 1-< 3 mm and ≥ 3 mm) as described (Moreno *et al.*, 1991). The

Table 2.6 : Body and Liver Weights of the Different Groups of Rats at the end of the Study (20 weeks) - 2 -stage Morphometry

Group	*No. of rats*	*Final body weight (g)*	*Liver weight (g)*	*Relative liver weight (g liver/100 gm body weight)*
A	10	285.7[a]±20.7	15.7±3.2	5.49±0.37[b]
B	10	310.5±25.1	10.5±3.0	3.38±0.20
C	10	298.8±26.2	10.99±2.18	3.64±0.32[c]
D	10	311.2±24.6	10.51±1.8	3.92±0.32
E	10	305.8±25.7	11.88±2.7	3.99±0.35
F	10	299.6±26.0	9.87±1.90	3.29±0.26
G	10	282.9±30.5	11.99±2.83	4.19±0.37
H	10	302.6±27.3	11.00±2.00	3.72±0.35

[a]Each value represents the mean±SE.

[b]P<0.02 as compared to group B.

[c]P<0.05 as compared to group A.

Table 2.7 : Effect of $CHCl_3$ Extract of *T. portulacastrum* on the Development of Hepatocyte Nodules in Livers of Rats Initiated with DENA and Promoted by Phenobarbital (P.B.)

Group	*No. of rats with nodules /total number of rats*	*Nodule incidence (%)*	*Total number of nodules*	*Average number of nodules/nodule bearing liver (nodule multiplicity)*
A	10/10	100	418	41.8±6.7[a]
C	3/10	30[b]	17	5.66±1.5[c]
E	6/10	60.0	140	23.3±3.9[d]
G	7/10	70.0	253	36.14±5.1

[a] Each value represents the mean ± SE.

[b]P < 0.001 as compared to group A by Fisher's exact probability test.

[c] P < 0.001 as compared to group A by students t-test.

[d]P < 0.001 as compared to group A by students t-test.

nodule incidence %, total number of nodules, and nodule multiplicity were calculated (Table 2.7). From the measured diameters, individual nodule volumes and nodule volume as percentage of total liver volume were calculated (Table 2.8).

Table 2.8 : Chemopreventive Role of $CHCl_3$ Extract of *T. portulacastrum* on the Size Distribution and Growth of Hepatocyte Nodules in Rats, Initiated with DENA and Promoted by P.B.

Group	No. of rats with nodules/ total no. of rats	Nodules relative to size ≥ 3 mm	<3- >1 mm	≤ 1 mm	Mean nodular volume[a] (cm^3)	Nodular volume/ liver volume[b] (%)
A	10	180	120	118	1.56±0.29[c]	62.1±5.8
C	3	3	6	8	0.62±0.11[d]	33.7±3.2[e]
E	6	35	32	34	0.91±0.15	51.7±5.3
G	7	39	28	33	1.22±0.20	60.2±5.8

[a] Individual nodule volumes were calculated from 2 perpendicular diameters on each nodule.

[b] 1 gm liver was assumed to occupy 1 cm^3 for this calculation.

[c] Each value represents the mean±S.E.

[d] P < 0.01 compared to group A by students t-test.

[e] P < 0.001 compard to group A by students t-test.

Table 2.9 : Effect of $CHCl_3$ Extract of *T. portulacastrum* on the Induction of Hepatic Foci in Rats, during DENA-PB Hepatocarcinogenesis

Group	No. of foci/ cm^2	Focal area (mm^2)	% area of liver parenchymia occupied by foci (%)
A	30.8±4.1	0.52±0.07	9.71±0.52
C	5.9±0.4[a]	0.26±0.01[a]	6.33±0.32[b]
E	16.0±2.5	0.33±0.06	7.40±0.46
G	21.3±3.1	0.42±0.05	8.0±0.57

Each value represents the mean ± S.E.

[a] P < 0.001, [b] P < 0.05 compared to group A.

For histological slides, thin sections of excised liver slices from right, left and caudate lobes of each liver, were dissected out and quickly immersed in 10% neutral buffered formalin. Embedded liver tissues were microtomed (5 μm thick) and stained with haematoxylin and eosin. Histological slides were scanned in different planes under a photomicroscope for specific hepatocellular lesions. Altered hepatocyte foci were counted (no/cm^2) and their number and size in mm^2, were calculated in different groups according to published criteria (Moreno *et al.*, 1991). The exact percentage area of liver parenchyma occupied by focal lesions, was also taken into consideration (Table 2.9).

2.6 Statistical Analysis

Statistical analysis for the hepatocyte lesions, in the different groups was performed by Fisher's exact probability test. All other data were analysed by student's t-test (Tables 2.6, 2.7, 2.8, 2.9).

3. Results

3.1 Food and Water Intakes

During the entire period of study, there was no treatment related observation, in the daily intake of food water.

Mortality

All animals survived during the entire course of the experiment.

3.2 Body and Liver Weights of the Experimental Animals

Table 2.6 depicts the final body weights of animals in grams, liver weight also in grams and relative liver weights of the animals sacrificed on the 20th week following DENA administration. There was a decrease in the final body weight of rats, subjected to DENA (carcinogen) alone, as compared to the normal control group. Treatment with $CHCl_3$-extract of *T. portulacastrum* raised the final body weights of the animls as evident in the Groups C, E and G compard to Group A. (carcinogen control). Liver weights were quite uniform in all the groups. The relative liver weights in Group A animals was significantly high in comparison to Group B animals (normal control); $P<0.05$. Again in Group C animals that received $CHCl_3$ extract of *T. portulacastrum* L. throughout the study (20 weeks), $P<0.05$ compared to Group A. (DENA control group).

3.3 Persistent Hepatic Nodules (PNs)

Supplementation of chloroform extract of *T. portulacastrum* to the animals, resulted in significant inhibition of DENA induced PB promoted hepatocarcinogenesis, and this was evident by the remarkably low nodule incidence (Table 2.7). There were no visible PNs in the livers of normal untreated rats (Group B) as well as in all the conrol Groups D, F, H. Significantly lowered $P<0.001$ incidence of PNs were observed in Group C that received the chloroform extract throughout the study, compared to Group A. In Group E where the extract was administered for only 4 weeks (initiation study as well as Group G, where the extract was administered for 15 consecutive weeks (promotion phase) also demonstrated a reduction of nodule incidence, in comparison to Group A. The result is statistically significant.

Of the three Group ie C, E, G, Group C showed maximum reduction in terms of nodule incidence %, total number of nodules, and nodule multiplicity. Nodule multiplicity in Group C, $P<0.01$ compared to Group A. In Group E also it was significant $P<0.05$ compared to Group A. Table 2.8 demonstrates the size distribution of PNs and depicts the mean nodular volume and also nodular volume as percentage of liver volume, among the different rats belonging to the Groups A, B, C, E, G.

The administration of chloroform extract of *T. portulacastrum,* characteristically reduced the appearance of PNs, greater than 3 mm in size in the Groups C, E and G, compared to Group A. In Group C mean nodular volume of 0.62 cm^3 was statistically significant. $P<0.01$ compared to Group A by student's t-test. In Group C nodular volume as percentage of liver volume is 33.7. Here $P<0.001$ compared to Group A by student's t-test.

3.4 Altered Hepatocyte Foci

Table 2.9 summarises the effect of the chloroform extract of *T. portulacastrum,* on the induction of hepatic foci in rats, during DENA PB hepatocarcinogenesis. In Group C the number of foci/ cm^2 was drastically reduced, $P<0.001$ compared to Group A. Here the focal area in mm^2 was substantially reduced, $P<0.001$ compared to Group A. In Group C the percentage area of liver parenchyma, occupied by foci was 6.33. This is statistically significant, $P<0.05$ compared to Group A.

3.5 Liver Histology of Rats Subjected to the DENA-PB Regimen

Altered hepatocyte populations were observed in the Groups A, E, G with variations in degree of alteration of liver cells. In

Group C the recovery was so great, that it approached the histologic profile of normal rats.

In H&E stained liver sections, focal changes were readily discernable from the surrounding normal parenchyma. In rats of Group A there was gross alteration of hepatocellular architecture. Phenotypically altered hepatocyte populations, appeared in the form of altered cell foci and nodules. Foci and nodules were much enlarged, assumed oval shape, trabeculae were drastically reduced. Nuclei showed marked degenerative changes and were largely vesciculated. Some nuclei were hyperchromatic with central nucleoli. Group B animals i.e. normal untreated controls, revealed normal central vein and portal tracts. There were radiating cords of polygonal cells, each with centrally located nucleus. Trabeculae were interspersed with sinusoids.

In animals belonging to Group C supplementation of the chloroform extract of *T. portulacastrum* L. during the entire course of the study, elicited maximum protection against DENA induced PB promoted hepatocarcinogenesis, as reflected in the nearly normal hepatocellular architecture.

In Group E a moderate improvement in the hepatocellular architecture was evident, in comparison to Group A. In the promotion phase (Group G) some improvement in the hepato-cellular phenotype from Group A was observed. Oval cells were observed in all DENA-treated groups A, C, E, G but no such alterations were observed in the control groups B, D, F and H.

In Group A animals, extensive vacuolation was observed in the cytoplasm, around the nucleus with masses of acidophillic material. Group C animals showed a preponderance of clear cell foci. Cells were filled up with cytoplasmic contents, with little or no signs of vacuolation. Group E animals displayed also a predominance of clear, rather than acidophillic cell foci, as was observed in the case of Group A animals. Vacuolation was less compared to Group A animals. In Group G, improvement of hepatocellular architecture was evident, but not so remarkable as that of animals belonging to Group C.

4. Discussion

The chemopreventive action of the chloroform extract of *Trianthema portulacastrum* appears to be mediated through inhibition of altered liver cell foci and hepatic nodule growth during the early stages of neoplastic transformation.

The findings indicate that in the 2-stage model of rat hepatocarcinogenesis, administration of the plant extract at a dose of 100 mg/kg body weight to the diet, of each animal once daily before initiation and during promotion, greatly reduced the incidence, multiplicity, and size of visible preneoplastic nodules along with an arrest of the number and dispersion of hepatic foci in the total liver parenchyma. The anticarcinogenic potential of the chloroform extract of *T. portulacastrum* was mainly observed in the initiation phase and secondarily in the promotion phase. However continuous treatment with the extract, could offer greater protection, in terms of magnitude of pre-neoplasia, than exposure at either initiation or promotion phase alone.

In the 2-stage model employed in the study, the extract when administered throughout the experiment, led to fewer rats developing visible PNs and smaller number of nodules per nodule bearing rat liver, than the Group A animals. Another fundamental observation in this study was that the extract inhibited the apperance of nodules, greater than 3 mm in size, with subsequent reduction of nodular volume, along with nodular volume as a percentage of liver volume.

It is however known that not all hepatocyte nodules become cancerous during the life span of animals; numerous observations support the concept that nodules are precursors of hepatic cancers (Farber, 1980; Williams, 1980).

There is a large body of observational experience in experimental and human disease, correlating the number and size of nodular hyperplasia and epatocarcinoma (Farber and Cameron 1980; Farber, 1990). There is also ample evidence indicating that hepatic preneoplastic lesions are putative precursors of hepatocellular carcinoma in rats and humans (Pitot *et al.*, 1980; Farber *et al.*, 1980). In view of this, inhibition of nodule growth and enhancement of their regression, with the chloroform extract of *T. portulacastrum,* is most crucial in cancer chemoprevention since PNs are easily discernable and are endowed with the capacity to regress spontaneously.

The food and water intakes and the body weights of the experimental animals were quite uniform. This proves that the chloroform extract is not toxic and fairly well tolerated by the animals. This has relevance because nutritional deprivation, causing weight loss, may parallel a decrease in the tumour volume (Waitzberg *et al.*, 1989). Perhaps it may be assumed that the inhibitory effect of the plant extract on nodule appearance and growth is not likely to be mediated by impairment of nutritional status of the experimental animals.

The role of the chloroform extract of *T. portulacastrum* in reducing the number of foci per cm^2 of liver area is evident from Table 2.9. The progressive loss of growth capacity by putative preneoplastic cells and their differentiation into nearly normal hepatocytes proceeds to a greater extent in presence of this active fraction of the plant *T. portulacastrum.* In the view of Pitot (1989), the number and size of altered liver cell foci, indicate initiating and promoting activities respectively. In this study, a decrease of focal area as percentage of liver area, were considered and the extract could remarkably slow down the growth of altered liver cell foci. This effect of the extract on focal growth, perhaps indicates selective toxicity to proliferating cells, since they are proliferating compared to a relatively non-proliferating backdrop, and thus slowly suppresses liver tumorigenesis.

The data were further susbtantiated by histological findings, which have shown that livers of chloroform extract supplemented rats (mainly Groups C and E) revealed near normal hepatocellular architecture with reduced structural regularities than the Group A rats.

DENA and other nitrosoamines confer carcinogenic action, through their metabolic activation generating DNA-binding alkylating agents (Swenberg, 1991).

Thus it may be concluded that rat liver carcinogenesis may be related to modification of metabolic activation and/or detoxification of the carcinogen involved, and the choloroform extract of *T. portulacastrum* has proved remarkable in inhibiting rat liver carcinogenesis mainly that initiated by DENA and promoted by P.B. Further the extract may play a role in remodelling the damaged tissue to the near normal state.

3

Antioxidant Defence and Hepatic Biotransformation Patterns in DENA-induced Rat Hepatocarcinogenesis Following Supplementation with *T. portulacastrum* Extracts

1. Introduction

The anticarcinogenic potential of the various fractions of *Trianthema portulacastrum* against a defined model of experimental hepatocarcinogenesis was undertaken, to assess the chemopreventive efficacy of the extracts with special reference to antioxidant defence and biotransforming enzymes in rat hepatocarcinogenesis. Since the process of carcinogenesis is accompanied by profound changes in the levels of glutathione and hepatic biotransformation enzymes, the study was designed to enlighten us on the role of these exracts in modulating the above markers. The liver has a paramount role in the metabolism of a wide variety of xenobiotics (Micozzi *et al.*, 1985; Wattenberg, 1985; Mayskens, 1988). The liver tissue was preferentially selected for the study because first liver is the target tissue for the site-specific hepatocarcinogen DENA. Second many chemical changes of the liver are detectable prior to the onset of secondary physiological and nutritional changes associated with pathological conditions such as neoplasia.

Third pathological changes in the liver often act as an indicator of overall damage caused by DENA, since liver enzymes provide more sensitive indicators of pathogenesis than blood (Herzfeld and Greengard, 1977). It was therefore thought worthwhile to investigate, as to how, the different fractions of the medicinal plant *Trianthema portulacastrum* can modulate hepatic xenobiotic detoxification and associated cellular defence mechanisms in rat.

Table 3.1 : Some Antioxidants in the Biological System

I	Enzyme antioxidants
	Catalase (CAT)
	Superoxide dismutase (SOD)
	Glutathione peroxidase (GPX)
II	Non-enzymatic regenerative antioxidants
	α-tocopherol
	Reduced glutathione (GSH)
III	Non-enzymatic exhaustable antioxidants
	Ascorbate
	β-carotene
	Uric acid
	Bilirubin
IV	Proteins sequestering
	Copper and Iron atoms
	Ceruloplasmin
	Ferritin
	Albumin

1.1 Antioxidant Enzymes

Antioxidant enzymes serve as a major cell defence against acute O_2 toxicity. Their function is to protect the membrane and other cytosolic components against damage caused by free radicals. Catalase, superoxide dismutase and glutathione peroxidase are classical enzymes of this group. Cells are constantly exposed to oxidative stress. Gene regulatory mechanisms within the cells, are able to recognize this oxidative stress, and induce overproduction of antioxidant enzymes, capable of reducing reactive oxygen species (ROS). They can in addition repair oxidative damage. Superoxide dismutase catalyses the conversion of O_2 to H_2O_2 (FridoVich, 1983). This is eventually destroyed by catalase enzyme, or by Glutathione peroxidase or Glutahione reductase (Gaettani *et al.*, 1989). GP_x and G.R. brings about the reduction of H_2O_2 to H_2O at the expence of NADPH, using GSH as e^- donor. Glycolytic enzymes regenerate NADPH. Some of the important antioxidants in the biological system are shown in table 3.1.

1.2 Hepatic Biotransformation Enzymes

Hepatic biotransformation enzymes are also known as drug metabolizing enzymes. This class of enzymes, catalyse the detoxification and excretion of foreign chemicals such as drugs and environmental pollutants. Being non-polar in nature, they dissolve quite easily in the lipid.

Hepatic biotransformation enzymes exert their catalytic activity, by converting these toxic chemicals into water soluble products, that are easily eliminated from the system. Enzymes, thus involved in drug metablism are classed into 2 types–Phase I and Phase II. Phase I enzymes are primarily concerned with functionalization process. Eg : Cytochrome P-450, the co-binding pigment of the liver microsomes. Phase II enzymes are involved in conjugation reactions. Eg : UDPGT.

Sato (1989) has stated that drug metabolising (hepatic biotransforming enzymes) are important markers in characterizing the metabolic patterns of pre-neoplastic cells. They are useful in the development of strategies for prevention of carcinogenesis and early treatment of cancer.

The Danger from Free Radicals

Glover (1990): "Free radicals refer to a group of molecules, possessing unpaired electrons, that can initiate/promote cancers". Reactive molecules are generated, by loss or gain of electrons (Halliwell and Gutteridge, 1989). The superoxide anion (O_2^-), a reduced oxygen species, is involved in acute oxygen toxicity. O_2^- dismutates to H_2O_2 and dioxygen. This step is catalysed by superoxide dismutase.

$O_2^- + O_2^- + 2H^+ \rightarrow H_2O_2 + O_2$

H_2O_2 in the presence of O_2 and Fe (III) or Cu (II) forms a hydroxyl (OH^-) radical (Halliwell and Gutteridge, 1989; Liochev and Fridovich, 1994).

H_2O_2 induces mutations, chromosome deletions, single stranded breaks, DNA protein cross links, thymine glycol adducts and other types of DNA damage (Imlay and Linn, 1988).

Nitric Oxide (NO$^{\cdot}$) is yet another physiological free radical (Moncada *et al.*, 1993; Bechman *et al.*, 1994). (Fig. 3.1).

1.3 Mechanism of Free Radical-mediated Injury

A : Frequently two free radicals happen to come together, unite by their unpaired electrons and establish a covalent bond.

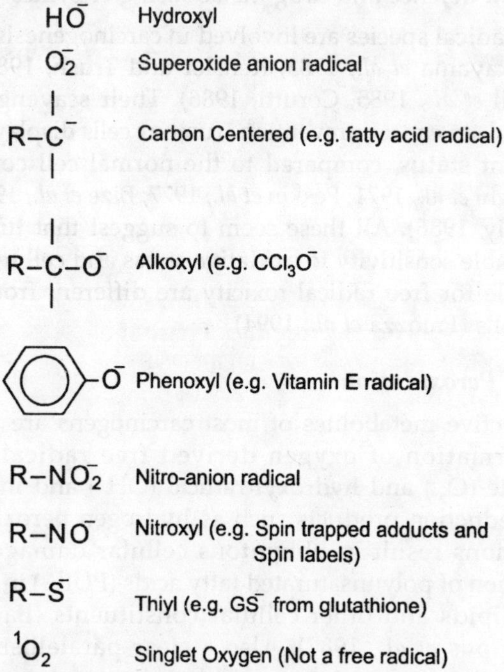

Fig. 3.1 : Free Radical Species that have been Implicated in a Wide Variety of Types of Tissue Damage Including Cancer.

$$\underset{\text{Superoxide anion}}{O_2^-} + \underset{\text{Nitric Oxide}}{NO^*} \longrightarrow \underset{\text{Peroxynitrite}}{ONOO^-}$$

Peroxynitrite at physiological pH, damages protein, and decomposes into toxic products.

B: Radical-Non-radical Interaction

Sometimes a free radical reacts with a non-radical, generating a free radical chain reaction evolving more and more new radicals.

Partially reduced species of oxygen are refered to as "reactive oxygen species" (ROS). These damage DNA and cellular entities and are implicated in causing diseases such as stroke, alzheimer's disease, emphysema, rheumatoid arthritis etc. (Gutteridge, 1988).

In view of the acute danger from free radials, it is imperative to study the enzymes involved in the detoxification process viz. antioxidant defence and drug metabolising enzymes.

Free radical species are involved in carcinogenesis (Tso *et al.*, 1977; Nakayama *et al.*, 1983; Kensler and Trush, 1984; Cerutti, 1985; Troll *et al.*, 1985, Cerutti, 1986). Their scavengers play a privotal role in cancer prevention. Tumour cells display abnormal antioxidant status, compared to the normal cell counterparts (Mochizuchi *et al.*, 1971; Peskin *et al.*, 1977; Bize *et al.*, 1980; Oberly and Oberly, 1986). All these seem to suggest that tumour cells have variable sensitivity to oxidative stress and cell mechanisms responsible for free radical toxicity are different from those of normal cells (Palozza *et al.*, 1994).

1.4 Lipid Peroxidation

The active metabolites of most carcinogens are thought to evoke formation of oxygen derived free radicals, such as superoxide (O_2^-) and hydroxyl radical (OH^-) and intermediate oxygen-reduction products such as hydrogen peroxide (H_2O_2). Their actions result in ubiquitous cellular damage, through peroxidation of polyunsaturated fatty acids (PUFA) in membrane phospholipids and other cellular constituents (Bacher *et al.*, 1982; Kappus *et al.*, 1987). Also a clear paralellism between carcinogenicity of a given xenobiotic and amount of active radicals generated has been found to exist (Slaga *et al.*, 1981; Goldstein *et al.*, 1981). Lipid peroxidation appears to be a common devastating consequence of oxygen free radicals (Esterbauer, 1982; Smith *et al.*, 1982).

Lipid peoxidation is a normal biochemical process, which involves the oxidation of polyunsaturated fatty acids (PUFA's) as components of cell membranes. Elevated lipid preoxidation in tissues has been associated wth tissue injury, due to generation of reactive species, which causes damage to cellular macromolecules, including DNA. *In vitro* and *in vivo* studies have shown that oxidation of PUFA's produce among other reactive compounds, a host of aldehydes (Esterbauer, 1990; WuH, 1995).

Enals of variable alkyl chain lengths Eg: trans-4-hydroxy-2-nonenal (HNE) arises from the oxidation of W-6-fatty acids like linoleic acid and has been detected in tissues of rodents at the estimated level of 8 n moles/g tissue (Esterbauer, 1991). Lipid peroxidation is involved in the endogenous formation of exocyclic adducts (Chung *et al.*, 1996).

Poly unsaturated fatty acids are very much susceptible to peroxidation and once initiated, the process, proceeds as a free radical chain reaction.

Agents bringing about the process have the ability to abstract a hydrogen atom from a methylene carbon in the side chain (Fig 3.2). The hydrogen atom is a free radical and its removal leaves behind an unpaired e^- in the C-atom, to which it was originally attached. The resulting carbon centred radical (L*) has several fates, but mostly it undergoes molecular rearrangement followed by reaction with oxygen to give a peroxyl radical, strictly under aerobic conditions. They are also capable of abstracting hydrogen atom, from adjacent fatty acid sidechains, in a membrane and thus propagates the chain reaction of lipid peroxidation (Kappus, 1987).

There are several reports of the deleterious effects of lipid peoxidation. These include enzyme inactivation, depletion of cofactors, formation of degradation products, some of which are chemical reactive and mutagenic *per se* (Marnett *et al.*, 1980; Ames *et al.*, 1982; Hammad *et al.*, 1990). The process causes impairment of membrane functioning (Slater *et al.*, 1971; Gutteridge, 1989) altered fludity, inactivation of membrane bound receptors. Lipid hydroperoxides have the ability to decompose upon exposure to Iron and Copper ions (Gutteridge, 1988; Gutteridge and Halliwell, 1989; Gutteridge, 1993). Lipid peroxidation causes lethal cell injury by liberation of hydroxy alkenals, particularly hydroxy-nonenal, which is a potent cytotoxin (Streeter *et al.*, 1984). Lipid peroxidation is a delayed event, accompanying rather than causing inevitable cell death (EKlow Lastbom *et al.*, 1986; Cochrane *et al.*, 1988). Cell and tissue destruction can lead to more lipid peroxidation, because antioxidants are diluted out and transition metal ions, that can stimulate the peroxidation process are released from the disrupted cells. Further an excellent correlation exists, between covalent binding of electrophillic species to tissue proteins and tissue necrosis (Boobis *et al.*, 1989) (Fig 3.2).

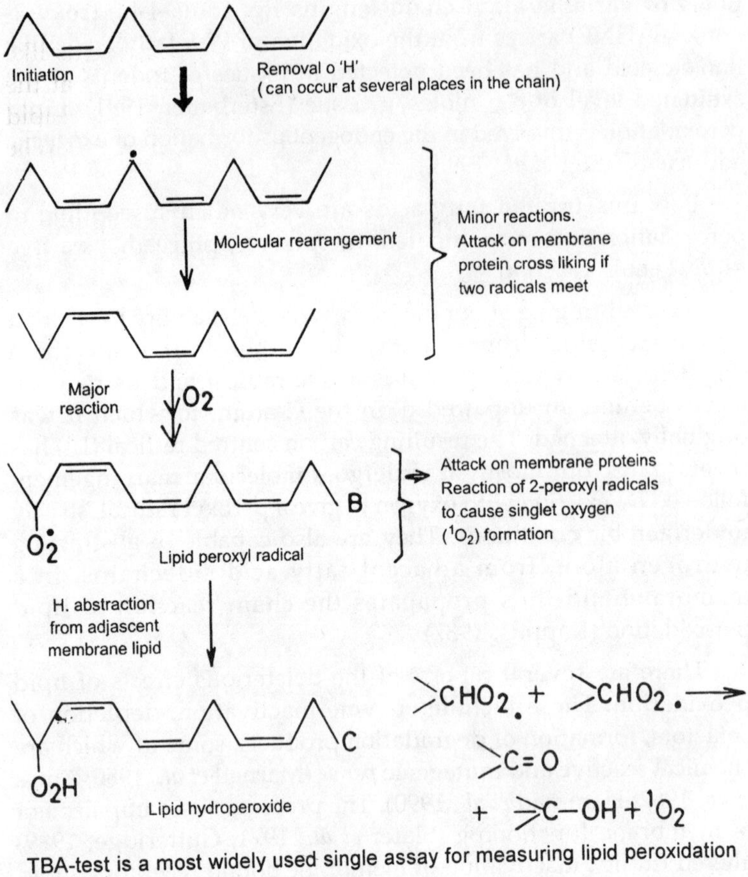

Fig. 3.2 : Schematic Representation of Lipid Peroxidation*.

1.5 *Glutathione*

The intracellular redox balance of mammalian cells is maintained by homeostatic mechanism, that links small pools of coenzymes and cofactors to a large redox buffer (i.e. thiol system with common chemical properties). Most of the extracellular and

---

* (Abstraction of hydrogen from a fatty acid with 3 double bonds is shown. A, B and C have conjugated–diene double–bond structures (double bond–single bond–double bond) that absorbs uv light at or around 234 nm).

intracellular thiols, is represented by the tripeptide glutathione, which is present in very high concentrations i.e. 2-10 m mols/litre (Uhlig and Wendel, 1992). Although both GSH and GSSG occur in tissues, GSH is by far the most predominant form. Greater than 99.5% of tissue total glutathione (i.e. GSH+GSSG, in GSH equivalents) is in the form of GSH. GSH readily oxidises non-enzymatically and it is a good substrate for γ-glutamyl transpeptidase (Andersson *et al.*, 1985). GSH is synthesized in the cells in a 2-step reaction involving A.T.P. The major control point in the synthesis is Reaction 1 i.e. γ-glutamyl cysteine synthetase reaction. This is subject to retroinhibition by GSH. This may be partially checked by an excess of glutamate that blocks the regulatory site on the enzyme (Meister, 1982; Meister and Andersson, 1983).

Inhibition of GSH synthetase (Reaction 2) leads to an accumulation of γ-glutamylcysteine, which in turn gets converted to cysteine and oxyproline under the catalytic influence of γ-glutamylcyclotransferase (Reaction 5). Oxoproline converts to glutamic acid by a 5-oxoprolinase reaction (Reaction 6). The relative levels of GSSG and GSH are regulated by a series of reactions (Reaction 9, 10, 11, 12).

In normal situations, the balance of the equation is far in the direction of maintaining cellular GSH and its reduced state. But when there is rapid production of GSSG (by reactions 11 and 9 and when glutathione reductase activity is imparied, GSSG seems to accumulate (Bannai 1984; Jen Kinson, 1987).

Breakdown of GSH is initiated by GGT, which catalyses the transfer of the γ-glutamyl Group of GSH and other γ-glutamyl compounds to acceptor molecules (aminoacids, dipeptides, GSH, H_2O etc.) (Reaction 3). Cystinyl glycine formed in the transpeptidase reaction, is split by dipeptidases to produce glycine and cysteine (Reaction 4) (Fig. 3.3). Glutathione acts as a reducing agent and an antioxidant and acts as a reservior of cyteine, participating in detoxification reactions for xenobiotics, and metabolism of numerous cellular compounds. Glutathione is involved in the synthesis of prostaglandins, and plays a major role in cell cycle regulation and thermotolerance (Parker *et al.*, 1980; Shaw and Chow, 1986; Furukawa *et al.*, 1987). It protects against tissue damage, resulting from exposure to oxidising environments, such as hyperoxia, hyperbasic oxygen or ozone (*De Lucia et al.*, 1975; Connor and Wheeler, 1987). It protects against radiation damage (Miller *et al.*, 1986). Intermediates produced during detoxification of xenobiotics, via glutathione transferase reaction, have been implicated in carcinogenesis (Deneke *et al.*, 1989).

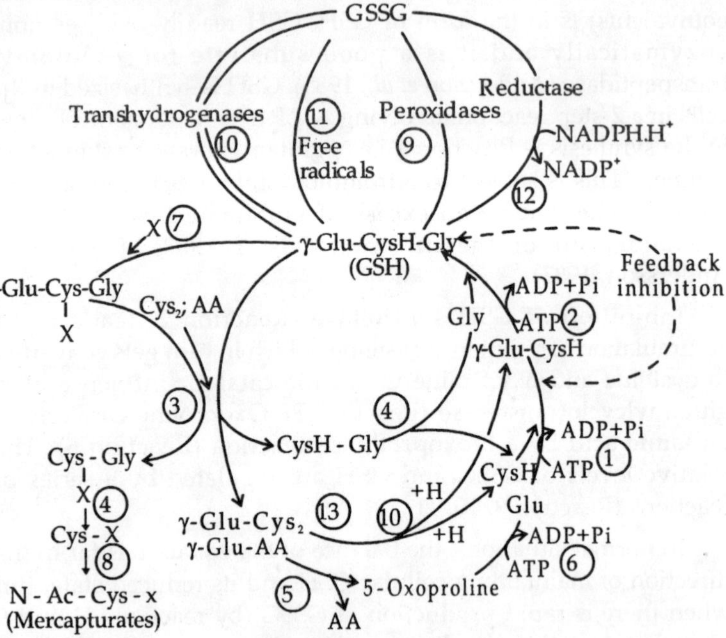

AA : Amino acids
X : Compounds that react with GSH to form conjugates
R1 : γ-glutamyl cysteine synthetase
R2 : GSH-synthetase
R3 : γ-glutamyl transpeptidase
R4 : Dipeptidases
R5 : γ-glutamylcyclotransferase
R6 : 5-Oxoprolinase
R7 : Glutathione-S-transferases
R8 : Glutathione
R9 : Glutathione peroxidases
R10 : Glutathionethiol-transferases
R11 : Reaction of free radical with glutathione
R12 : Glutathione disulphide reductase
R13 : Transport of γ-glu $(cys)_2$.

Fig. 3.3 : Outline Biochemistry of Glutathione.

1.6 GSTs

Glutathione S-transferases are thought to play a physiological role in initiating the detoxification of potential alkylating agents (Booth *et al.*, 1961; Boyland *et al.*, 1969; Wood *et al.*, 1970). This includes pharmacologically active compounds. GST's catalyse, the reaction of compounds with -SH Group of glutathione, and thus neutralizes their electrophillic sites and renders the products more water soluble. Glutathione conjugates are thought to be metabolized further by cleavage of the glutamate and glycine residues followed by acetylation of the resultant free amino group of the cysteinyl residues to produce the final product mercapturic acid (Boyland *et al.*, 1969, Habig *et al.*, 1974). Thus excretion of mercapturate and CH_3-S-CH_3-SO-$CH_3SO^-_2$ containing metabolites are indicative of the *in vivo* formation of GST-conjugates of xenobiotics. Mercapturic acids are then excreted. GST's were identified by Booth *et al.*, 1961 in rat liver and have subsequently been purified. GST's are a family of multifunctional proteins, which act as enzymes, and also as binding proteins in various detoxification processes (Jakoby *et al.*, 1980; Mannevick, 1985; Ketterer, 1986). Toxic products generated from tissue damage of reactive alkenes, epoxides, hydroperoxides, arachidonic acid (Tan *et al.*, 1986; Danielson, 1987) are substrates of GST. In addition, 4-hydroxyalkenals, the cytotoxic and mutagenic products of membrance lipid peroxidation are also substrates of GST enzymes (Totter, 1980; Esterbauer, 1982).

GST binds with high affinity several hydrophobic compounds, like polycyclic aromatic hydrocarbons and dexamethasone (Litwack *et al.*, 1971; Arias *et. al.*, 1976). Mouse liver GST's have attracted attention with regard to antioxidant associated chemoprevention of hepatocarcinogenesis (Benson *et al.*, 1979; 1884; Pearson, 1983; Wattenberg, 1986; Bock *et al.*, 1989).

GSTs have also been acknowledged as Preneoplastic and neoplastic markers (Sato, 1989). With respect to cancer, these enzymes probably 1) Protect normal cells from initiation by chemical carcinogens 2) If augmented during preneoplasia, they give preneoplastic cells, a selective advantage over neighbouring cells (Farber, 1984a; Manson and Ketterer, 1988; Hayes and Wolf 1988).

Several naturally occurring products and dietary constituents are known to induce GST activity, which has been correlated with their antineoplastic action (Wattenberg, 1992; Nijhoff *et al.*, 1993). Some dietary antioxidants with antitumour properties, raise GST activites (Benson *et al.*, 1978; 1979; Talalay, 1979; Sparnins *et al.*, 1982; Moorghen *et al.*, 1991). GSTs probably have a role in the protective mechanism against tumour development.

1.7 Cytochrome P-450 Monooxygenase

The presence in mammalian liver microsomes of a carbon-monoxide binding pigment has been reported (Klingenberg, 1958; Garfinkel, 1958). The co-compound of the reduced pigment, has an intense absorption band at 450 mμ and can thus be readily detected in dithionite treated microsomes by difference spectrophotometry. Chemically P-450s are haemoproteins in nature and can be converted into a solubilized form, termed P-420, by treatment of microsomes anaerobically with snake Venom or deoxycholate (Omura and Sato, 1964). P-450s are most numerous of all drug metabolising enzymes having a very broad range of substrate specificity both endogeneous and exogenous, including drugs, prostaglandins, steroids, chemical carcinogens and xenobiotics (Wislocki *et al.*, 1980; Guengerich, 1990). P-450 dependent enzymes, also known as mixed function oxidases carry out biotransformations ie CN-S-hydroxylations, dehalogenations, dealkylations, deaminations and reductions. It can metabolise numerous chemicals providing the basis for their collective capacity to metabolize and detoxify diverse substances, found in the diet and environment.

The P-450 gene superfamily encodes numerous enzymes, and so far about 150 have been characterized (Porter and Coon, 1991). Some P-450s are very specific in selection of substrates and those in the hepatic E.R., catalyse numerous chemical reactions, with an almost unlimited number of biologically occurring xenobiotic compounds (Black and Coon, 1987; Porter and Coon, 1991).

In mammals, P-450 has been found in several organs and the liver seems to possess the same in very high concentration (Bast and Haenen, 1984). A critical step in P-450 catalysed reaction is the formation of OH donor, which then transfers the OH Group to the appropriate position on the substrate. The overall reaction catalysed by P-450's proceeds with the stoichiometry.

$$RH+O_2+NADPH+H^+ \rightarrow ROH+H_2O+NADP^+$$

Here RH denotes the substrate. The product is ROH as shown in the Fig. 3.4.

Cytochrome P-450 content in hepatocytes shows regional variations in normal and induced livers (Wattenberg *et al.*, 1972; Salmon *et al.*, 1974; Altman *et al.*, 1975). Cytochrome P-450, MC1 and MC2 species are markedly decreased in foci and hyperplastic nodules induced by DENA (Buchman, 1985). Cytochrome P-450 facilitates detoxification in some instances, and in others converts biologically inert compounds to harmful products. They may catalyse, metabolic activation of some substrates to highy reactive free radicals, alkyating or arylating agents that react with DNA/RNA to initiate toxic carcinogenic events (Guengerich, 1991 b). It is yet to be ascertained, that the complex nature of P-450s may detoxify and or/aid in the genesis of both acute and chronic liver cell injury (Gravela *et al.*, 1975; Paolini *et al.*, 1992).

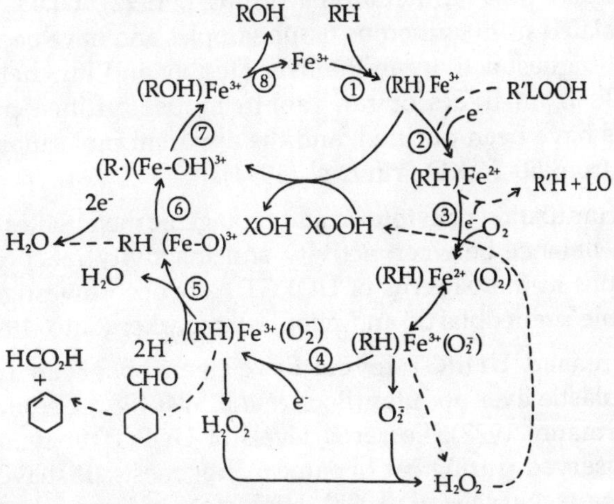

RH represents the substrate, ROH represents the corresponding mono-oxygenation product.

R'LOOH Lipid hydroperoxide.

R'H and LO (Corresponding reduction products i.e alkane and OXO acid).

XOOH Peroxy compound that serves as an alternative O_2 donor to molecular O_2.

Fig. 3.4 : Schematic representation of the mechanism of action of cytochrome P-450 enzyme system. Fe represents Haeme, iron atom in the active site.

1.8 UDPGT

UDPGT enzymes are a class of enzymes involved in glucuronidation, i.e. conjugation reaction, in the metabolism of xenobiotics (Tephly and Burchell, 1990).

The basic reaction that eventually proceeds to a glucuronide is R-OH-UDPGA →R-OGA+UDP.

Here ROH is the xenobiotic, UDPGA = UDP gluconic acid. This class of enzymes have broad overlapping substrate specificities in response to the need to eliminate potentially toxic endobiotic and environmentally produced xenobiotic compounds. UDPGTs catalyse the reaction of nucleophilles, such as phenols, amines, thiols, and carboxyllic acids with UDPGA, to yield polar and readily excretable products. These enzymes also provide a method for bioregulation of important endogenous hormones, bile acids and bilirubin (Dutton, 1980) UDPGT's are responsible for the excretion of potentially carcinogenic compounds (Dutton, 1980; Bock *et al.*, 1989). UDPGT's are membrane bound proteins, the highest activities are found in the E.R. membrane, particularly the smooth E.R., but appreciable activity is found in the nuclear and cellular plasma membrane (Mudler, 1992), UDPGTs have been isolated from numerous tissue samples and have been found to exert highest activity in the liver (Tephly and Burchell, 1990). UDPGTs from livers of rat, rabbit, mouse, guinea pigs and humans have been purified, and the apparent molecular weight ranges from 50-56 KD (Yin *et al.*, 1994).

Accumulation of cytotoxic and mutagenic metabolites depend upon a balance between activity and inactivity reactions. The alterations in the patterns of UDPGT have been investigated, as a possible preneoplastic and neoplastic marker (Sato, 1990).

Increased UDPGT levels have been observed in some preneoplastic liver nodules (Bock *et al.*, 1974; 1982; Gessner, 1977; Zimmermann, 1977). Lowered levels of UDPGT enzymes have been observed during rat hepatocarcinogenesis (Bishayee *et al.*, 1994; Bhattacharya *et al.*, 1998). High rates of lipid peroxidation probably lowers the levels of UDPGT in cancer cells.

The accumulating evidence suggests common factors of biochemical properties early in the development. Biochemical properties confers on the early new cell population a resistance to the cytotoxic effects of xenobiotics, that could play a privotal role in the carcinogenic process (Fidler and Hart, 1982; Woodruf, 1983).

Preneoplastic marker enzymes in rat liver can be divided into two groups–one demonstrating decreased activity and the other demonstrating increased activities. In general, enzymes and isoenzymes related specific hepatic functions are decreased in the foci. Cyt-P-450 enzymes are more numerous than all other bio transformation enzymes, with broadest substrate specificity (Wislocki *et al.*, 1980; Guengerich *et al.*, 1990). Cyt P-450 MC_1 and MC_2 species are markedly decreased in foci and hyperplastic nodules induced by DENA (Buchmann, 1985).

Cameroon *et al.*, (1976) observed a significant reduction in the concentration of cytochrome P-450 and aryl hydrocarbon hydroxylase in rat livers subjected to the carcinogen 2 AAF. AHH was reported to be decreased in the nodules during chemical hepatocarcinogenesis (Tsuda *et al.*, 1977; Cammeron and Sweeny, 1976).

GSTs are reliable markers for preneoplastic lesions and liver neoplasia. Isozyme forms of GST include rat placental form (GT-P or G-777 and the human placental form GT-II). Isoforms display similarities in physiochemical, enzymatic and immunological properties, and have thus been grouped together in class II under species independent classification of GST (Mannervick, 1985).

Several groups have investigated the changing GST isozymes in rat liver carcinogenesis and they show elevated trends (Sato, 1990; Kitagawa, 1983). GT-P has been identified as a good reliable marker for rat hepatic preneoplastic foci (Sato *et al.*, 1984; Meyer *et al.*, 1985; Pickett *et al.*, 1987). 3-5 fold rise in mRNA levels of GT subunits Ya/Ye and Yb_1/Yb_2 of hepatocyte nodules using complementary DNA and 30-fold increase of GST levels during early stage of rat hepatocarcinogenasis induced by SF model (1988) have been observed (Pickett *et al.*, 1984).

2. Materials and Methods

2.1 Plant Material

Dried plant sample was supplied by united allied plant products, Calcutta.

2.2 Extraction of Plant Material

Air dried, pulverized plant material of the whole plant (excluding roots) of *Trianthema portulacastrum* was subjected to extraction process using soxhlet's apparatus. The plant powder was first run through petroleum ether (to remove oils) and subjected to successive runs through benzene, chloroform, acetone and finally ethanol. Each time 2.5 litres of solvent was used for 225 g of pulverized plant material. 5 fractions of plant material were obtained. The pet-ether, benzene and acetone fractions were stored for future use. Only the EtOH and chloroform fractions were used for experimental purpose. Each fraction of the plant extract was subjected to distillation, then evaporated in vacuo and kept under refrigeration until used. Crude extract of the plant was prepared by refluxing the pulverized material in double distilled water (Devi and Ganasoundari, 1995).

Chemicals

Thiobarbituric acid, DENA, NADPH, UDPGT, UDP-glucose, CDNB, BSA, GSH were procured from sigma chemical company, St. Louis, U.S.A. All other chemicals were of high purity grade obtained from E. Merck, India.

Animals

Male Sprague Dawley rats weighing 110-120 g were obtained from Indian Institute of Chemical Biology (C.S.I.R.), Calcutta, India and were selected for the entire experiment. Animals were housed six rats per cage, in suspended, wire bottomed galvanized cages in rooms controlled for temperature (24±1°C) and relative humidity (50-60%) with 12 hour light/dark cycles and had free access to standard pellet diet (Lipton India) and water adlibitum during the entire experiment.

2.3 *Experimental Protocol – Treatment Schedule*

After initial acclamatization for a period of 10 days, the animals were divided at random into the following groups:

Experimental Regimen

Group A′	*Trianthema* Controls.
Group A	Normal Untreated Control
Group B	Carcinogen control (DENA treated)
Group C	Carcinogen + crude aqueous extract of the plant.
Group D	Carcinogen + EtOH extract of the plant.

Group E	Carcinogen + $CHCl_3$ extract of the plant.
Groups F and G	Served as EtOH control and chloroform extract controls respectively.

All rats in the experimental groups (except control animals and Group A animals) were administered DENA in 0.9% NaCl solution at a dose of 200 mgs/kg body weight (Ogawa *et al.*, 1980), intraperiotonialy (ip) to initiate carcinogenesis. Concomittent with carcinogen administration, treatment using different fractions of the plant extract was started, to identify the fractions, showing maximum response in each of the groups C, D, E. Plant extracts at a dose of 100 mg/kg body weight was added to the basal diet of each animal once daily. Control animals of Group A', F and G also received the extract at the same dose ie 100 mgs/kg body weight.

2.4 *Preparation of Microsomal and Cytosolic Fractions*

Prior to biochemical estimation, animals were fasted overnight, and sacrificed under light either anaesthesia. Samples of each liver lobe were promptly excised, washed in chilled normal saline, blotted and weighted. All subsequent operations were carried out at 0-4°C. Livers were homogenized individually in ice cold 0.154 M KCl using a teflon glass homogenizer (5 strokes) to yield a 10% w/v homogenate. The homogenate was centrifuged at 9000xg for 20 minutes using a Sorvall SS-34 rotor. The supernatant obtained was further centrifuged at 105000xg for 60 minutes, in an OTD-50B Sorvall Ultracentrifuge at 4°C. The supernatant obtained through this second centrifugation formed the cytosolic fraction, the pellets, were resuspended in the homogenizing medium and served as the microsomal fraction.

2.5 *Biochemical Assays*

Hepatic (cytosolic) lipid peroxidation was determined by the method of Ohkawa *et al.*, (1979), which is based on the formation of Malone-dialadhyde (MDA).

Microsomal lipid peroxidation were estimated according to the method of Hammad *et al.*, (1990) by incubating the microsomal suspensions with NADPH, and the samples were assayed for TBARS production. The TBARS were measured in mgs/microsomal protein in the assay.

Ellman's method (1959) was used for the estimation of the amount of GSH in 1 ml of cytosol. GSH was mixed with 1 ml of 4% 5-sulfosalicylic acid. The mixture was centrifuged at 1500xg for 15 minutes and the supernatant was allowed to react with 0.1 mM 5,5-dithio-bis (2-nitrobenzoic acid). The solution was then kept at room temperature for 10 minutes and read at 412 nm by a shimadzu uv-3000 spetrophotometer. Results were expressed as μmols of GSH/g of wet tissue.

The activity of cytosolic GSH-t was measured by the method of (Habig *et al.*, 1974) using CDNB or DCNB and GSH as substrates. The reaction mixture 1 ml consisted of 0.1 M Potassium Phosphate buffer (pH 6.5), 1 mM GSH, 1 mM CDNB or (0.5 mM DCNB) and a suitable amount of cytosol (1.0-1.5 mg protein/ml). The reaction mixture was incubated at 37°C for 5' and the reaction was initiated by addition of CDNB or DCNB. The increase in optical density at 340 nm was measured spectrophotometrically. Specific activity of GSH-t was expressed as μ moles of GSH-conjugate formed/min/mg of protein. Protein content both cytosolic and microsomal were assayed according to the method of Lowry *et al.*, (1951) using BSA as the standard.

Cytochrome P-450 content was measured in the microsomal fraction by method of Omura and Sato (1964), using Sodium dithionate and co-saturated water. Cytochrome P-450 was measured spectrophotometrically at 450 nm.

Table 3.2 : Effect of the Extract (s) of *T.portulacastrum* L on Hepatic Cytosolic GSH-content of Rat Liver in DENA Induced Hepatocarcinogenesis

Group	*Treatment*	*GSH content in μ moles/g tissue*	*S.E.*
A'	Trianthema control	4.75	± 0.26
A	Normal control	4.70	± 0.24
B	DENA control	9.30⁺	± 0.44
C	DENA + Crude aqueous extract of T.P.	6.15*	± 0.17
D	DENA + EtOH extract of T.P.	6.73*	± 0.33
E	DENA + $CHCl_3$ extract of T.P.	4.98*	± 0.33

Each value represents the mean ± SE of six animals,

⁺ P<0.001 with respect to Group B,

* P<0.001 with respect to Group A.

Table 3.3 : Effect of the Extract(s) of *T. portulacastrum* on Hepatic Cytosolic GSH-t Content of Rat Liver in DENA Induced Hepatocarcinogenesis

Group	*Treatment*	*GSH-t content in (μ moles GSH- conjugate produced/min/mg protein)*	*S.E.*
A'	Trianthema control	1.50	± 0.22
A	Normal control	1.52	± 0.16
B	DENA control	2.72+	± 0.19
C	DENA + Crude aqueous extract of T.P.	1.85**	± 0.19
D	DENA + EtOH extract of T.P.	1.89**	± 0.19
E	DENA + $CHCl_3$ extract of T.P.	1.67**	± 0.22

Each value represents the mean ± SE of Six animals,

\+ P<0.001 compared to Group A,

** P<0.01 compared to Group B.

Table 3.4 : Effect of Extract(s) of *T. portulacastrum* L on Hepatic Microsomal Cytochrome P-450 Monooxygenase in DENA Induced Rat Hepato Carcinogenesis

Group	*Treatment*	*Cytochrome P-450 content in (n moles/mg protein)*	*S.E.*
A'	Trianthema control	0.60	± 0.02
A	Normal control	0.63	± 0.03
B	DENA control	0.30+	± 0.02
C	DENA + Crude aqueous extract of T.P.	0.52*	± 0.01
D	DENA + EtOH extract of T.P.	0.48**	± 0.02
E	DENA + $CHCl_3$ extract of T.P.	0.58*	± 0.03

Each value represents the mean ± SE of six animals,

\+ P<0.001 compared to Group A,

** P<0.01 compared to Group B,

* P<0.001 compared to Group B.

Table 3.5 : Status of Hepatic Cytosolic Lipid-peroxidation in DENA Induced Rat Hapatocarcinogenesis After Treatment with Extracts of *T.portulacastrum.*

Group	*Treatment*	*n moles of MDA/ gm of tissue*	*S.E.*
A'	Trianthema control	2.29	± 0.20
A	Normal control	2.36	± 0.37
B	DENA control	7.56⁺	± 0.47
C	DENA + Crude aqueous extract of T.P.	3.31*	± 0.20
D	DENA + EtOH extract of T.P.	5.86***	± 0.41
E	DENA + $CHCl_3$ extract of T.P.	2.80*	± 0.21

Each value represents the mean ± SE of six animals,

⁺P<0.001 compared to Group A,

* P<0.001 compared to Group B,

***P<0.05 compared to Group B.

Table 3.6 : Status of Hepatic Microsomal Lipid Peroxidation in DENA Induced Rat Hepatocarcinogenesis Subjected to Treatment with Extracts of *T. portulacastrum* L.

Group	*Treatment*	*(n moles of TBARS/ mg of microsomal Protein*	*S.E.*
A'	Trianthema control	3.40	± 0.31
A	Normal control	3.41	± 0.41
B	DENA control	14.26⁺	± 0.36
C	DENA + Crude aqueous extract of T.P.	4.85*	± 0.31
D	DENA + EtOH extract of T.P.	6.24*	± 0.36
E	DENA + $CHCl_3$ extract of T.P.	3.80*	± 0.23

Each value represents the mean ± SE of six animals,

⁺P<0.001 compared to Group A,

*P<0.001 compared to Group B.

Table 3.7 : Effect of *Trianthema* Extracts on Hepatic Microsomal UDPGT Levels in Rat Liver Tissue in DENA Induced Hepato Carcinogenesis

Group	*Treatment*	*n moles of glucuronide/ min/mg protein)*	*S.E.*
A'	Trianthema control	23.66	± 0.82
A	Normal control	23.86	± 0.96
B	DENA control	9.89+	± 0.55
C	DENA + Crude aqueous extract of T.P.	19.39*	± 0.42
D	DENA + EtOH extract of T.P.	16.83*	± 1.06
E	DENA + $CHCl_3$ extract of T.P.	22.05*	± 0.71

Each value represents the mean ± SE of six animals,

+ P<0.001 compared to Group A,

* P<0.001 compared to Group B.

Microsomal UDP-glucuronyl transferase (UDPGT activities, towards 4-nitrophenol (4-NP) and phenolphthalein (PPT) were assayed by the method of Watanabe *et al.*, (1986) (Tables 3.2, 3.3, 3.4, 3.5, 3.6, 3.7).

3. Results and Discussion

The results of our present study have shown that the chloroform extract of *Trianthema portulacastrum* L. is more potent than the other plant fractions in restoring glutathione status to near control values in experimental hepatocarcinogenesis (Tables 3.2 and 3.3). (Bhattacharya *et al.*, 1998).

Hepatic biotransformation enzymes have also been strongly influenced by the chloroform extract of *Trianthema portulacastrum* L. (Tables 3.4 and 3.7). The extract further was remarkable in maintaining near control levels of lipid peroxidation (Tables 3.5 and 3.6) (Bhattacharya *et al.*, 1998).

From epidemiological as well as experimental studies, it has been shown that isolation and exploitation of naturally occurring secondary metabolites, as inhibitors of carcinogenesis from plants, offers great promise for obtaining chemopreventive agents effective in loweing the incidence of cancers in humans (Loub *et al.*, 1975; Pantuck *et al.*, 1976). An enormous range of dietary constituents of plant origin, have been reported to inhibit neoplastic transformation in experimental animals (Benson *et al.*,

1984; Wattenberg *et al.*, 1984; Hussain *et al.*, 1990; Janu *et al.*, 1991). Reactive oxygen species (ROS) play an important role throughout the carcinogenesis process especially during the promotion stage (Deflora, 1990; 1991). Antioxidants inhibit carcinogenesis when administered either prior to or concommitant with carcinogen administration (Novi, 1981; Ames, 1983).

Intracellular effects of carcinogens are inhibited by modulating their passage through the cell membrane either by preventing their uptake or by favouring the elimination of conjugated metabolites out of the cell.

Trapping and detoxification of xenobiotics provides the organism with an important defensive mechanism impairing the potential carcinogenicity of these substances (Benicelli *et al.*, 1985; Deflora *et al.*, 1978).

Single DNA adduct was observed in the liver of wister rats, subjected to 2 AAF. Co-administration of antioxidant NAC in the diet, resulted in the decrease in this adduct formation (Teebor and Becker, 1971).

Synchronous fluorescence spectrophotometric studies (SFS) showed that antioxidants have the power and ability to remove adducts upon administration (Vahakangas *et al.*, 1985).

Certain mechanisms such as antigenotoxic, and antioxidant activities have relevance also in the later steps of carcinogenesis. GSH has been shown to prevent tumour promotion (Perchellet *et al.*, 1985; and progression; Roltstein *et al.*, 1988).

Prevention or delay of cancer in experimental animals provides a convincing endpoint for assessing the anticarcinogenic properties of putative inhibitors, and for predicting their protective efficacy in human subjects. GSTs are a class of detoxification enzymes, which catalyse the reaction of GSH, one of the major endogenous antioxidants, with numerous electrophillic sites, including activated forms of chemical carcinogens, to yield less toxic conjugates readily excretable (Chasseaud *et al.*, 1979; Jakoby *et al.*, 1980). The excretable products contain exceptionally stable thioether linkage (Wattenberg, 1983).

In the biochemical assays involving hepatic cytosolic GSH and hepatic cytosolic GSH-t-activities, Group B animals (carcinogen control group) displayed marked increase in the levels of cytosolic GSH and GSH-t contents. The *Trianthema portulacastrum* treated groups, most notably Group E animals showed near normal levels of GSH and GSH-t-indicating clearly the chemopreventive efficacy of the extract against tumourigenic insult (Marnett and Turtle, 1980; Yonei and Furni, 1981). The enhancement of GST/GSH has been noted in Group B animals. The exact mechanism by which the extract maintains near normal levels of GSH/GST in extract treated groups in unknown. It is possible that the plant extract inhibits the metabolic activation of the carcinogen, with strong antioxidant and free radical scavenging activity.

MDA the product of lipid peroxidation has been known to be carcinogenic (Basage, 1989). Increased lipid peroxidation in cancerous processes is likely to aggravate the neoplasia. GSH protects the liver cell against lipid peroxidation (Christopherson, 1968; Haenan and Bast, 1983) by inhibiting free radical formation (Bast and Haenen, 1989). This increase of GSH, GSH-t contents in Group B animals, maybe viewed as an attempt by the host-cells to prevent DNA damage which occurs in the carcinoma from oxidative stress (Halliwell and Gutteridge, 1989). The increased levels of these enzymes may perhaps also afford protection from components of the immune system (Reiners *et al.*, 1991).

GGT levels increase in chemical rat hepatocarcinogenesis (Fiala *et al.*, 1972) GGT catalyses the degradation of extracellular GSH and is perhaps involved in the production of precusors, that can be used in the intracellular synthesis of GSH (Reiner *et al.*, 1991). Closer investigation reveals that cystenyl glycine, the cleavage product of GSH by GGT is a potent mutagen, that gives rise to a thiolate anion (Stark *et al.*, 1988). This damages tissue by generating ROS (Glatt *et al.*, 1990; Uhlig and Wendel, 1992). Thus elevation of GSH levels in Group B animals may be pictured as an attempt by the host cells to combat the existing oxidative stress. The extract was unique as it could effectively tackle the onslaughts imposed by DENA.

Lipid peroxidation being an auto-catalytic free radical process is much accelerated in Group B animals (Table 3.5). In Lipid Peroxidation poly unsaturated fatty acids (viz linoleic acid, arachidonic acid, docosahexanoic acid in the bio membranes get degraded to water soluble short chain carbonyl compounds

(Beneditti *et al.*, 1979; Dillard and Tappel, 1979; Esterbauer *et al.*, 1982) and to lipid hydroperoxides which decompose to yield epoxy-fatty-acids, alkenes, alkanals, alkenals, L_1-hydoxyalkenals and aldehydes (Slater, 1984; Esterbauer, 1985).

Peroxidation of lipids has been implicated as a general mechanism for destruction of cell membrane integrity due to alterations in fluidity, fall in membrane potential, increased permeability to H^- and the other ions eventually leading to rupture and release of cells and organelle contents (Fong *et al.*, 1973; Gutteridge, 1993). Lipid Peroxidation levels on the rise have also been noted in the pathogenesis of several cardio vascular, pulmonary and hepatic neuronal diseases and also during ageing. (Comporti, 1985; Poli *et al.*, 1987; Yagi, 1991).

The formation of lipid endoperoxide in unsaturated fatty acids, leads to the formation of MDA as a breakdown product (Pryor *et al.*, 1978). In Group C animals (treated with crude aqueous extract of *Trianthema portulacastrum*). Lipid peroxidation levels were not too high but in Group E animals lipid peroxidation levels were closely resembling, the normal values, indicating the strong chenopreventive efficacy of the extract in checking pathological cell injury. The highly enhanced levels of lipid peroxidation in the liver tissues of Group B animals indicates, the strong membrane damaging effects of DENA in the Group administred DENA alone. Decreased levels of lipid peoxidation in all the extract treated groups seems to suggest, the potential of the extract to act as a blocking agent, in experimental hepatocarcinogenesis.

In the second experiment of lipid peroxidation (Table 3.6) involving microsomal lipid peroxidation in hepatic tissues of rat, TBARS has been used as index for measurement of the extent of lipid peroxidation. NADPH dependent microsomal lipid peroxidation is known to be mediated by ADP/Fe^{2+}, NADPH - Cyt P-450 reductase and Cyt P-450 (Cajelli *et al.*, 1987). So a fall in the levels of these modulators in the liver may be the possible explanation for reduced lipid peroxidation levels in all the *Trianthema portulacastrum* extract treated groups, more specially in Group E. Reduced rates of lipid peroxidation may perhaps be due to free radical trapping agents and/or significant decrease of PUFA by the extract (Svinger *et al.*, 1979). The apparent inhibitory effect of the extract on lipid peroxidation suggests that possibly the extract inhibits infiltration of inflammatory cells and/ or releases the action of reactive oxygen species from these cells.

A relative deficiency of cytochrome P-450 levels in hyperplastic nodules have been observed in case of 2 AAF treated rat liver (Cameron *et al.*, 1976). In the experiment using DENA, Cyt-P-450 levels were drastically reduced on the 22nd week, following carcinogen administration (Table 3.4) (Group B). Low levels of Cyt-P-450s have also been reported for various other hepatomas (Conney *et al.*, 1967; Hagihara *et al.*, 1973; Oyanagui *et al.*, 1974).

In the other experimental groups C, D, E cytochrome levels were much higher and in Group E animals treated with $CHCl_3$ fraction of *Trianthema portulacastrum*, Cytochrome P-450 levels were high, showing beyond doubt, the ability of the fraction to bring about tough resistance against the necrogenic effect of DENA. *Trianthema portulacastrum* L. was more than capable in bringing the levels of the Phase I enzymes, to near normal levels. It is possible that the plant extract inhibits the binding of metabolites to DNA. This inhibition of metabolic activation occurs via Cyt-P-450 enzymes along with the induction of other detoxifying enzymes.

The marked decrease in the activity of UDPGT enzyme (Phase II) in Group B animals compared to Group A was observed (Table 3.7). This may be taken to mean, an overall failure of the detoxification process under the necrogenic effect of DENA. However *Trianthema portulacastrum* mediated maintenance of UDPGT activity in all *Trianthema portulacastrum* treated Groups C, D, E more notably Group E reflects the important role of the extract in accelerating the glucuronidation reactions. This is perhaps effected through the induction of UDPGDH activity, thereby providing more UDP glucuronic acid to be utilized by the enhanced UDPGT activity.

Since glucuronic acid conjugation is catalysed by the conjugation enzymes joining the Phase I metabolites (often more toxic) to an endogenous conjugating agent forming more water soluble derivatives that are eliminated from the body (Merill and Bray, 1982), hence a decrease in UDPGT activity is probably due to the necrogenic effect of DENA (Newmann and Zannoi, 1990a,b) or due to inefficient elimination of potentially toxic compounds (Tephly Burchell, 1990). UDPGT is a tightly bound microsomal enzyme, sensitive to changes in protein-lipid interaction (Zakim, 1988; Castuma and Brenner, 1989). It is not clear as to how the folded enzyme interacts with the phospholipid phase of the membrane, (Mudler, 1992). Therefore slightest perturbation in the membrane can cause severe inactivation of the enzyme in question. An enhanced lipid peroxidation has been observed in Group B animals and therefore it is likely that the alteration in the membrane environment is affected resulting in disaggregation of UDPGT and a reduction in its catalytic activity. Reduction in UDPGT activity is probably due to the availability of UDP-glu-A which in turn depends upon glycogen as a spare capacity. When glycogen is depleted (fasting condition) the availability of UDP-glu - A is decreased, leading to an inhibition of glucuronidation (Gregus *et al.*, 1990).

Thus inhibition of UDPGT activity upon exposure to carcinogen has a correlation with decreased glycogen levels, produced since the animals were fasting.

In the other experimental Groups C, D, E UDPGT levels were much like the expected normal levels more so in the case of Group E animals treated with chloroform extract of *T. portulacastrum*. A lowering of the levels of UDPGT enzymes in rat hepatocarcinogenesis has been reported earlier from our laboratory (Bishayee *et al.*, 1994). A correlation between inhibition of carcinogenesis and microsomal oxidation and cytosolic detoxification have been reported (Cha *et al.*, 1979; Wattenberg *et al.*, 1984).

So in view of the correlation seen between chemoprevention of chemical carcinogenesis and microsomal oxidation and detoxification, the extract was able to modulate, the enzyme activities of both Phases I and II of drug metabolism and antioxidant defence.

The induction of Phase II enzyme activities as for Phase I activities, increases the detoxification of some chemicals but at the same time, increases the bioactivation of many others (Paolini *et al.*, 1992). So considering the double action of xenobiotic metabolising enzymes, from a toxicological point of view each metabolising component of either Phase I or II should be considered as an activating-detoxifying system. It depends on the nature of the chemical reaction catalyzed (Paolini *et al.*, 1995).

Inducers of cytochrome P-450 enzymes and Phase II inducers, are prospective anti-initiating agents that have been employed in experimental models, for inhibitng experimental tumour initiation (Morse and Stoner, 1995).

Nevertheless GSTs are still known to detoxify far more carcinogens than they activate. Epidemiologic studies have revealed that cruciferous vegetables, plant herbs, etc. which induce GST in animals and human being prevent cancers (Morse and Stoner, 1995).

However the best way to understand the anticarcinogenic effects of dietary substances, plant extracts etc. is to assume that they act additively or synergistically. This is plausible because extracts contain many substances that may act on the same or different steps of carcinogenesis (Vang *et al.*, 1997).

4

Influence of the Various Extracts of *T. portulacastrum* L. on Hepatic Histology and Histochemistry Against DENA-Induced Rat Liver Carcinogensis

1. Introduction

Hepatic tumours induced in rats by prolonged exposure to large doses of the potent carcinogens are usually multiple, numerous and uniform in size as though they developed simultaneously. Multiple tumours are evenly distributed throughout the different lobes of the liver. However some observers believe that the liver right lobe, notably the upper portion, serves as a locus of predilection for the development of tumours and tumours in the right lobe are very much prone to metastatise (Griesemer *et al.*, 1980).

Histologic typing of liver tumours in rat is designed to provide uniform categorization of tumours. It helps to promote comparability in the assessment of the results of experiments on liver carcinogenicity and of bioassays of potential or suspected environmental carcinogens. Histologic sections stained with Haematoxylin and Eosin, enables us to get a proper insight into the tissue level changes/alterations brought about by the carcinogenic insult, from gross findings at necropsy, and other features of the lesions present. The study was intended to observe the changes brought about by subsequent treatment by the different fractions of *Trianthema portulacastrum*, including the activity of the crude aqueous extract of the plant.

In the present study other methods were employed to study features such as mucopolysaccharide, reticulin to understand the changes induced by DENA, in experimental carcinogenesis, coupled with the chemopreventive ability of the extract to repair tissue damage following treatment.

The rationale behind the selection of these parameters lies in the fact that at least some changes in glycogen status and pattern of fibrosis are found during carcinogenesis, but none is due to specific effects of carcinogens (Kimbrough *et al.*, 1975; Bannasch *et al.*, 1976).

2. Materials and Methods

Plant Material

Dried overground parts of the plant *T. portulacastrum* L. were supplied by United Chemical and Allied Products, Calcutta, India. The plant was authenticated by the Botanical Survey of India, and a voucher specimen number (Ju/Pharm/Biochem/SPO3) has been deposited in the same herbarium.

2.1 Extraction of the Plant Material

Air dried overground parts of *T. portulacastrum* L. were crushed in a crusher and the fine pulverized material was subjected to extraction in a soxhlet's extractor with Pet-ether (b.p. 60-80°C). The pet-ether extract was discarded. The marc was extracted successively with benzene, chloroform, acetone, and finally ethanol 95% w/v (Vohra *et al.*, 1983). The chloroform and alcohol extracts were subjected to distillation, evaporated in vacuo, and the material contained 4.6% w/w and 4.8% w/w of the extracts in a highly concentrated form. Crude aquous extract was prepared by refluxing the fine pulverized plant material in double distilled water (Devi and Ganasoundari, 1995). Prior to plant drug administration to the experimental animals 0.2 ml of 0.05% Tween 80 were added to the chloroform fraction of *T. portulacastrum* in double distilled water to enhance solubility of the fraction in water.

Animals

Male Sprague Dawley rats, weighing 110-120 g were obtained from Indian Institute of Chemical Biology (C.S.I.R.), Calcutta, India and were selected for the entire experiment. Animals were housed 4 rats per cage i.e. 16 rats/group in suspended wirebottomed galvanized cages, in rooms, controlled for temperature (26 ± 1°C) and relative humidity (± 70%) with 12 hour light/dark cycles and had free access to standard pellet-diet (Lipton

India) and were supplied water adlibitum during the entire experiment.

2.2 *Experimental Protocol*

After initial acclamatization for about two weeks, the animals were divided at random into several experimental and control groups. Group A animals (16 animals) were the normal untreated controls. Group A′ animals were *Trianthema* controls, the Group B animals served as the carcinogen control group and received only DENA. Group C animals were administered DENA, followed by treatment with the crude aqueous extract of the plant *T. portulacastum* Group D animals also received the carcinogen, concurrent administration of EtOH extract of *Trianthema portulacasrum* L. was started in this group. Group E animals received DENA followed by subsequent tretment with the $CHCl_3$ extract of the plant.

All the experimental animals except animals of Group A, and A′, (Trianthema controls) were administered DENA in 0.9% NaCl solution at a dose of 200 mgs/kg body weight (Ogawa *et al.*, 1980), intraperitonially to initiate carcingenesis. In the Groups C, D and E treament was started the next day after carcinogen treatment, following a 24-hour recovery period from stress, after i.p injection of DENA. Group C animls were fed crude aqueous extract of the plant at a dose of 100 mgs/kg body weight once daily. The same dose was applicable to the other groups (experimental and controls) treated with the different plant fractions (EtOH and $CHCl_3$ fractions). Treatment was continued for 22 weeks. Animals were sacrificed on the 22nd week under light ether anaesthesia.

2.3 *Histologic and Histochemical Evaluation*

Representative liver pieces, were scissored from the left, right, median and right anterior liver lobes and quickly immersd in 10% neutral buffered formalin. Following fixtion, the tissue slices were processed further for paraffin embedding.

After fixation in 10% neutral buffered formalin the tissues were thoroughly dehydrated by passing through a series of progressively increasing concentrations of alcohol with one change in each concentration, and a duration of one hour in each case. Absolute alcohol was changed three times (Mukherjee 1988).

After dehydration of the tissue samples, removal of alcohol was accomplished by using xylene, the clearing agent, to make the tissues ready for infiltration and impregnation.

In the next step, after clearing, the tissues were transferred to a bath of molten paraffin wax in an embedding oven for infiltration and impregnation. Infiltration and impregration, leading to the removal of xylene were carried out at 50-56°C for 2-3 hours in a paraffin oven.

Subsequent to infiltration and impregnation, the tissues were embedded in warm, low melting point liquid paraffin, and eventually solidifield into a firm block, within the Leuckhard embedding boxes housing them.

Sections of 5 μm thickness were obtained in the form of flat, ribbons in a rotary microtome and the ribbons were initially made to float on warm water in a shallow water bath at a constant temperature of about 46°C (10°C below the melting point of wax). Only the flat, fully expanded, un-distorted ribbons containing the embedded tissue were chosen, and removed carefully on slides using a camel hair paint brush.

Prior to routine histopathological evaluation by Haematoxylin and Eosin (H and E staining) the tissues were first deparaffinised in xylene, rehydrated by passing through decreasing grades of alcohol (i.e. absolute, 90%, 80%, 70%) and finally washed in distilled water.

2.4 Routine Haematoxylin and Eosin Staining Procedure

Haematoxylin is a natural dye obtained from the leguminous plant *Haematoxyln indica.* It is the principal stain for demonstrating the nucleus and cytoplasmic inclusions. It works in conjunction with alum which acts as a mordant. Alum containing haematoxylin stains the nucleus light transparent blue. The stain which is picked up by the cytoplasm, gets removed more rapidly than the nuclear stain, when treated with acid solution (differentiation). At this stage, the stain differentiates the nucleus and the cytoplasm. A second solution is required at this point to neutralise the acid solution. The counter stain used is Eosin, which is picked up by all tissues revealing the general structure.

Staining procedure was followed according to the method of Mukherjee *et al.,* (1988) and involved the following steps:

- First washed in running tap water, rinsed in distilled water, water allowed to drain off.
- Stained sections with Harris Haematoxylin for 7-10 minutes, washed in running tap water.
- Slides dipped quickly in and out of 0.5% HCl for 60 seconds in coplin jars.
- Washed in water-30 seconds.
- Dipped several times in dilute ammonia till section assumed a bluish coloration washed again.
- Rinsed in 95% alcohol.
- Agitated in Eosin staining solution for 10-60 seconds. Stain drained off after staining.
- Placed slides in 70% alcohol for 50 seconds.
- Placed slides in 95% alcohol for 50 seconds.
- Placed slides in absolute alcohol for 60 seconds, each having two changes.
- Cleared in xylene-60 seconds each-2 changes.
- Allowed excess xylene to drain off.
- Perfect sections, mounted on Canada balsam, covered with coverslip, and sealed for observation under a photomicroscope. Specific hepato cellular lesions were observed under light microscope according to published criteria (Bannasch, 1976; Stewart *et al.*, 1980).

2.5 *Histochemical Evaluation of Tissue Samples*

Histochemical techniques primarily periodic-acid-schiff reaction (PAS) and Reticulin pattern were incorported in the study to observe DENA-related changes in the different experimental groups, and the activity of the plant extract in modifying the changes in the glycogen status as well as fibrillar pattern of hepatocytes in chemical rat hepatocarcinogenesis.

The staining and identification of the various types of carbohydrates, poly and mucopolysaccharides have contributed greatly to our understanding of tissue structures like liver (glycogen), heart striated muscles, and GI tract glands. The use of PAS method in histology dates back to 1947 when Mc Manus demonstrated mucin and Schabadasch (1947) demonstratd glycogen (Pearse *et al.*, 1985).

Periodic acid is a strong oxidant which breaks the C–C bonds in various structures, where these are present as 1,2-diol groups (>C–OH_C<OH_). Converting them into carbonyl group (>C=OO=C<). Thus R-CHOH-CHOH-R′ -> R-CHO OHC-R′.

If incorporated in a ring system, the -OH groups of the glycol maybe either cis or trans to each other. The reaction proceeds with the following mechanism.

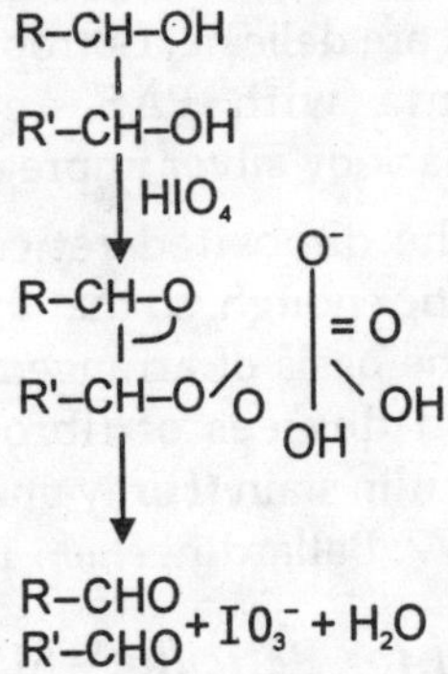

The α-hydroxy amino or alkyl aminostructures R-CHOH-CH (NHR-R′-R" are also converted to RCHO and R" CHO while α-hydroxyketones, R-CHOH-CO-R', are split to RCHO and R'CO_2H).

Periodic acid has a selective advantage over other oxidants such as $KMNO_4$, H_2O_2, H_2CrO_4 in that, it does not oxidise the resulting aldehydes and these can therefore be localized by combination with Schiff's reagent to give a subsituted dye which is rose-red or purple red in colour. An intense rose-red colour indicates positive PAS reaction.

2.6 Staining Protocol : PAS Reaction

- Deparaffinised sections rinsed in distilled water.
- Made to oxidise in 0.5% periodic acid for 8 mins-washed in running tap water for 3 minutes.
- Stained with Schiff's reagent for 15 minutes.
- Placed in running tap water for 10 minutes, for rose colour to develop fully.
- Stained with Harrishaematoxylin for 3 minutes and differentiated by means of 4 quick dips in 1% acid alcohol.

- Washed in running tap water till bluish colour forms.
- Dehydrated, cleared, mounted and observed under light microscope.

When haematoxylin is used as a counter stain, nuclei stain blue, PAS positive zones become rose coloured.

Reticulin (Puchtler, 1964) refers to a substance derived from reticulum fibres, after removal of their gelatin content. Reticulin consists of fibrillary extracellular framework in connective tissues. The fibrills of reticulin are delicate, isotropic and stains pink with Van Gieson, magenta with PAS, red with sulphation-metachromasia and black by silver impregnation (Pearse, 1985).

The pattern of the deposited reticulum in a tumour is sometimes characteristic enough, so that the origin of the tumour can be identified on the basis of arrangement of reticulin in the tumour. Further mild degrees of fibrosis in organs can be recognized by the reticulin stain (Hirayama *et al.*, 1970; Periano *et al.*, 1971; Solt *et al.*, 1977; Ballardini *et al.*, 1983).

2.7 *Staining Protocol for Reticulin – Silver Impregnation*

The staining was performed in coplin jars, and comprised of th following steps.

- Oxidised with potassium permanaganate (0.5%) for 2 minutes.
- Washed in tap water for 2 minutes.
- Bleached with 5% oxalic acid for 2 minutes until colour subsided.
- Washed in tap water.
- Sensitized with 4% $FeCl_3$ for 2 minutes.
- Washed in running tap water for 3 minutes.
- Washed thoroughly in distilled water.
- Allowed impregnation in silver solution for 1-5 minutes.
- Rinsed in distilled water for 20 seconds.
- Reduced for 3 minutes with formalin.
- Washed in tap water for 3 minutes.
- Toned in 0.2% Auric chloride solution for 10 minutes.
- Rinsed in distilled water.

- Fixed in 5% sodium thio-sulphate for 5 minutes.
- Washed in distilled water.
- Dehydrated, cleared, mounted in Canada Balsam and observed under photomicroscope. Reticulin fibres have an affinity for silver and stain black following impregnation with silver.

Chemicals

DENA was purchased from Sigma Chemical Co. (St Louis, Mo, U.S.A). All other chemicals were of analytical grade and obtained in the purest form unless otherwise specified.

3. Results

Histological changes of rat hepatocyte tissues were investigated. Histologial examination of liver sections of Group A animals i.e. those belonging to the normal untreated controls, revealed normal hepatic architecture (Fig. 4.1) comprising of radiating cords of polygonal cells, each with centrally located round nucleus. The cords appear to arise from the central hepatic vein. The normal liver parenchymal cells reveal granulated cytoplasm. The trabeculae are interspersed with sinusoids. The reticulin pattern is clearly normal, with nil signs of fibrosis (Fig. 4.2). PAS positive zones are as expected in normal tissues and seem to be housed within the inclusions seen within the heptocytes (Fig. 4.3).

Figs. 4.4 and 4.5 picture sections through the necrotic factor, (a while thread, with a head resembling a spatula) isolated from the preneoplastic nodule of the carcinogen control group (Group B). Histologic profile of the necrotic factor reveals a disorganized cellular architecture with pronounced degenerative changes. Dysplastic change was observed in the slides. Focal necrosis of the liver cell is clearly apparent and the cells in all the slides appear to possess hyperchromatic nucleus. There is marked fibropathy of tissues in between liver cells accompanied by eosinophillic and plasma cell infiltration. All sections show the presence of a cryptic body of unknown nature. Almost all nuclei are pyknotic, presenting a clumped apperance exhibiting a richly vacuolated state. Balooning degeneration, fatty changes were also observed. Fig. 4.6 reveals a section through the neoplastic nodule, in Group B animals (DENA control Group). The nodule showed degenerative changes but no dysplastic change was observed at all places. Focal necrosis was quite remarkable. In H&E sections of the neoplastic nodules, many types of altered hepatocytes were clearly distinguished. Clear cell areas, glycogen rich areas, ground glass cells presenting a whorled appearance, vacuolated cells with lipid droplets and cells with mixed clear and basophillic or mixed acidophillic and basophillic cytoplasm were observed. PAS positive zones were observed. Reticulin pattern was disrupted, typical of tumours (Fig. 4.7). There was chronic infiltration of infiltrate around the bile ducts, but not within the cell chords.

Fig. 4.8 depicts a section of hepatic tissue of Group B animals. H&E stained slides of this group (DENA control group) revealed a grossly altered heptocellular architecture, with phenotypically altered hepatocyte populations, in the form of altered liver cell foci and nodules. Hepatocytes were oval in shape, much enlarged, largely vesciculated and mosly binucleate in the foci and nodules. The nuclei appeared to be pyknotic, with kinky structure. The hexagonal liver lobule showed signs of positive atrophy and necrosis. Kupffer cell hyperplasia was prominent. There was extensive vacuolation in the cytoplasm, with masses of acidophillic material. In most of the slides, lymphocytic infiltration around the portal tracts and in between the cords of the hepatocytes were observed PAS positive areas were quite extensive (Fig. 4.9) and were stained deep rose coloured. Fig. 4.10 depicts a section through the liver tissue of rats, belonging to Group C (i.e. those animals treated with crude aqueous extract of the plant following DENA administration. Here no frank degeneration, necrosis or nuclear changes were observed. There was a definite improvement of the histopathological profile in that pyknosis was almost absent, binucleate cells were much reduced in number, foci were predominantly of clear cell type, vacuolation in the cytoplasm was much reduced. Only very mild kupfer cell hyperplasia and sparse lymphocytic infiltrate could be observed in the slides. Reticulin pattern closely approached the normal pattern. Hepatocytes showed near normal PAS positive inclusions within the cytoplasm (Fig. 4.11). Supplementation of the EtOH extract of the plant to the DENA treated animals (Group D) (Fig. 4.12) showed liver architecture within normal limits. There was mild periportal increase of reticulin fibres (figure not shown). Liver cells showed fewer PAS positive inclusions (Fig. 4.13) vacuolation was present but much reduced. Cytoplasm was still agranular with cell and nuclear pyknosis far less than the DENA control group. Clear cell foci were numerous but seemed to be intermingled with mixed and eosinophillic foci.

However supplementation with $CHCl_3$ extract of the plant to the Group E animals following a single ip injection of DENA, elicited maximum protection against the DENA induced hepatocarcinogenesis, as reflected in the nearly normal hepatocellular architecture (Fig. 4.14). The hepatocytes looked normal. There was absence of pyknosis, cell and nuclear size appeared to be normal blood vascularity was normal, binucleate cells were absent. A predominance of clear cell foci were noted. PAS positive zones were normal (Fig. 4.15). Reticulin pattern was also similar to the normal pattern, as found in Group A animals (Fig. 4.16). No signs of malignancy were observed in all the H&E stained slides of the Group E animals.

Control animals revealed tissue structures similar to Group A animals. PAS reaction reticulin pattern in the controls were similar to that of the untreated normal controls.

4. Discussion

In most of the models of hepatocarcinogenesis, focal areas of altered hepatocytes become grossly visible nodules that precede the appearance of malignant tumours. These preneoplastic lesions are considered to be the possible precursors of hepatic cancers in rat and may be humans as well (Farber and Cameron, 1980; Farber, 1990).

Treatment with several hepatocarcinogens results in the proliferation of oval cells. These cells can differentiate into hepatocytes or into ductular cells (Sell, 1990). Studies on the development of these cells during carcinogenesis indicate that liver cancer arises from oval cells (Sell, 1990).

Supplementation of the $CHCl_3$ fraction of the plant to the basal diet of the experimenal animals elicited maximum protection against DENA induced rat hepatocarcinogenesis which was reflected in the nearly normal hepatocellular architecture liver cells from this group were found to contain compact cytoplasmic material with only clear cell foci. The configuration of the sinuses appeared normal with normal kupfer cells. The nuclei appeared normal, with absence of degenerative changes. A moderate improvement of the hepatic histological picture was observed in Group C animals who were fed 100 mg/kg body weight, crude aqueous extract of the plant. Pyknosis was nearly absent, binucleate cells were drastically reduced in number. Foci were primarily of clear cell type, accompanied by a much reduced vacuolation of the cytoplasm.

The EtOH extract treated group, showed liver architecture within normal limits, with mild periportal increase of reticulin fibres and fewer PAS positive areas. Pyknosis was much less compared to Group B animals and there was an abundance of clear cell foci which however was found to remain intermingled with mixed and eosinophillic foci.

Chemically induced hepatic fibrosis in experimental animals has attracted a great deal of attention (Cameron *et al.*, 1963; Lieber *et al.*, 1974). Continuously occurring liver cell regeneration enhances the development of hepatocellular carcinoma (Wada *et al.*, 1996). In humans, chronic liver cell necrosis and compensatory regeneration, occurring during active viral hepatitis, is always accompanied by progressive fibrosis, intimately involved in promoting hepatocellular carcinoma development (Miyaji *et al.*, 1976; Borzi *et al.*, 1995). In terms of histolgical appearance, the livers of rats treated with swine serum (ss) exhibited an increase in fibrotic tissues of variable thickness, with bridge formation from portal area to portal area (-P bridging) and occasionally from portal areas to central regions of lobules (P-C bridging) producing pseudo lobule formation resembling cirrhotic conditions found in man (Wada *et al.*, 1996).

Reticulin is represented by fibrillar extracellular framework in connective tissues. The pattern of the deposited reticulin in a tumour indicates the origin of the tumour, and helps in the identification of characteristic tumours (Mukherjee, 1988).

In all the experimental Groups B, C, D, E reticulin pattern was studied. In Group A animals (normal, untreaed controls), and in Group A' animals (*Trianthema* control animals) the reticulin pattern was normal. Group B animals, displayed drastic changes in the pattern of reticulin fibrills as is characteristic of tumours with marked fibrosis.

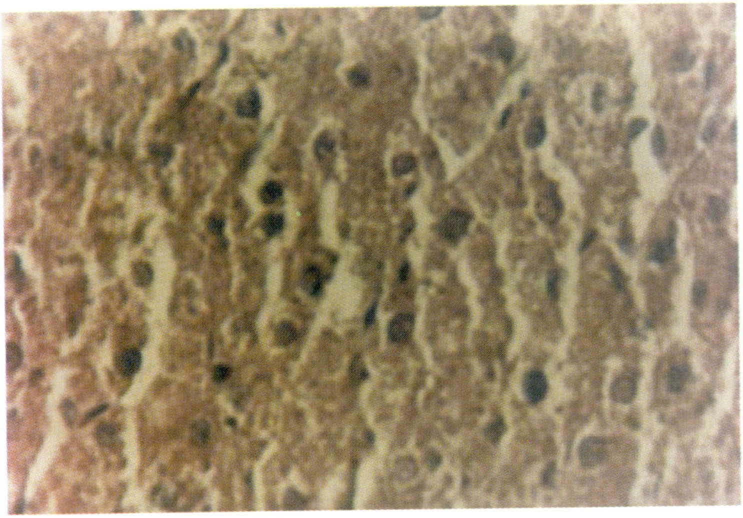

Fig. 4.1 : Thin section of liver of normal untreated rat showing normal hepatic architecture (H & E × 400).

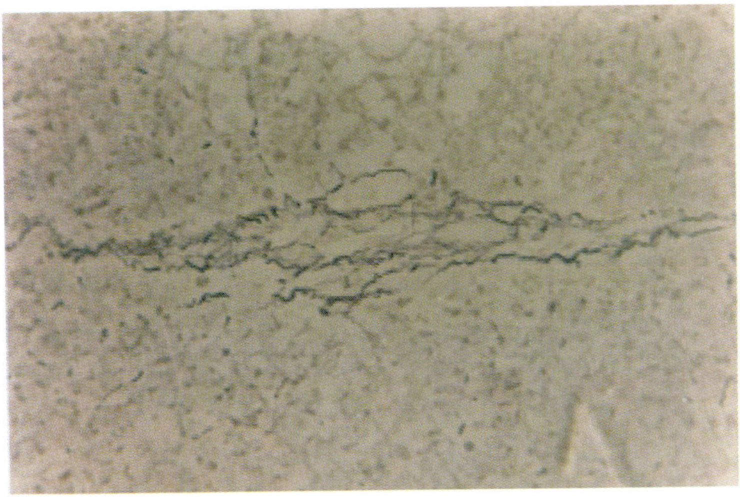

Fig. 4.2 : Normal arrangement of reticulin fibre in normal untreated rat liver (× 400).

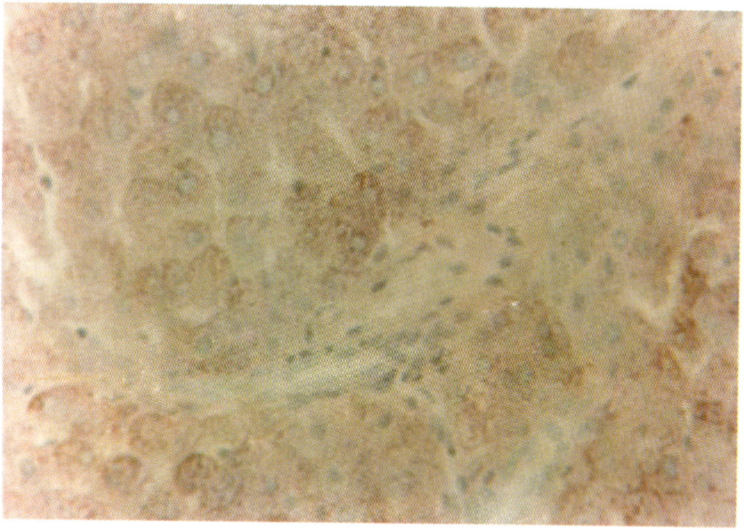

Fig. 4.3 : Thin section of normal untreated rat liver showing normal PAS reaction (× 400).

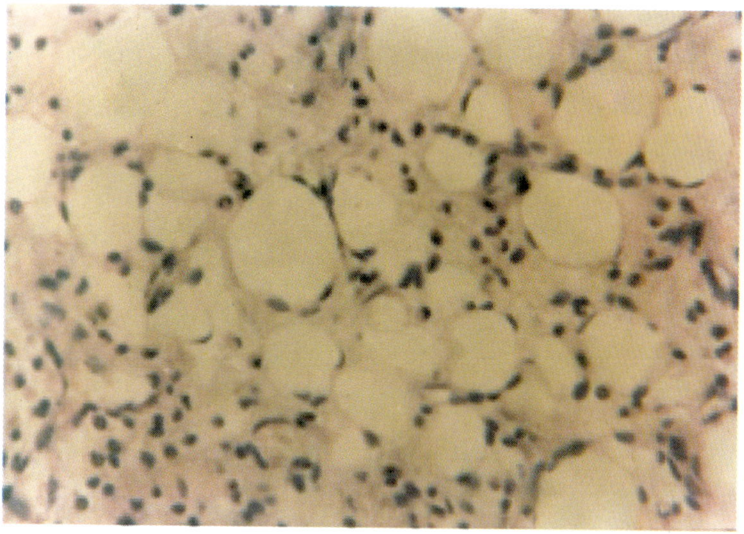

Fig. 4.4 : Section through the necrotic factor (H & E × 400).

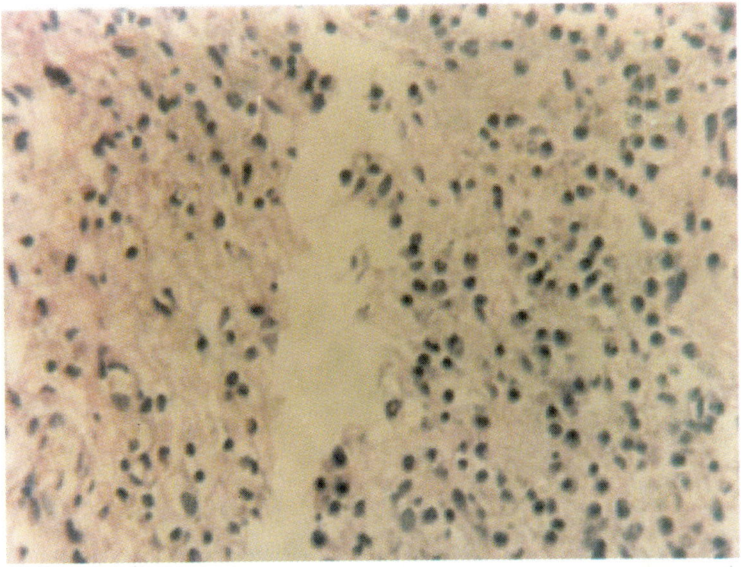

Fig. 4.5 : Section through the necrotic factor (H & E × 400).

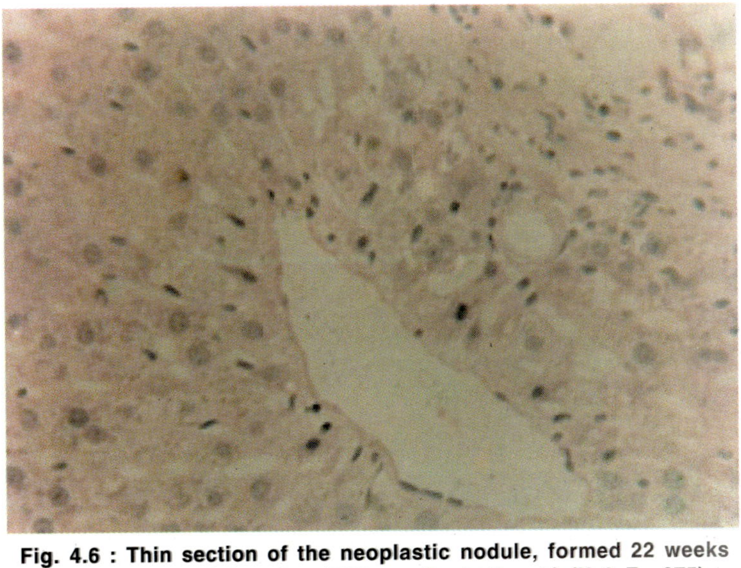

Fig. 4.6 : Thin section of the neoplastic nodule, formed 22 weeks after DENA administration (200 mgs/kg body wt.) (H & E × 275).

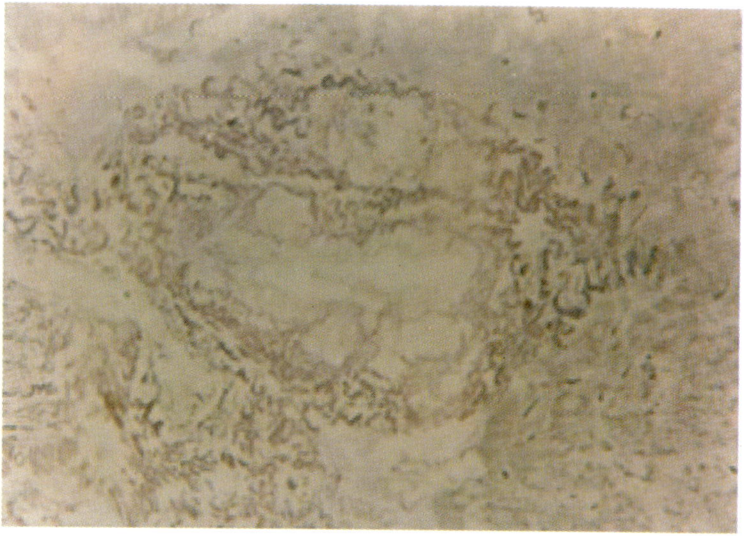

Fig. 4.7 : Section of rat liver depicting arrangement of reticulin in DENA control group (× 400).

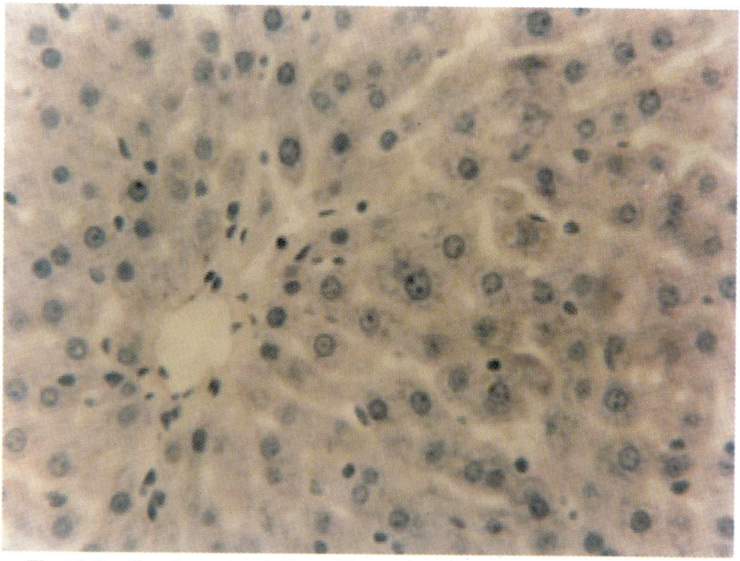

Fig. 4.8 : Section at rat liver 22 weeks after ip injection of DENA (200 mgs/kg body weight) showing abnormal hepatic architecture (H and E × 400).

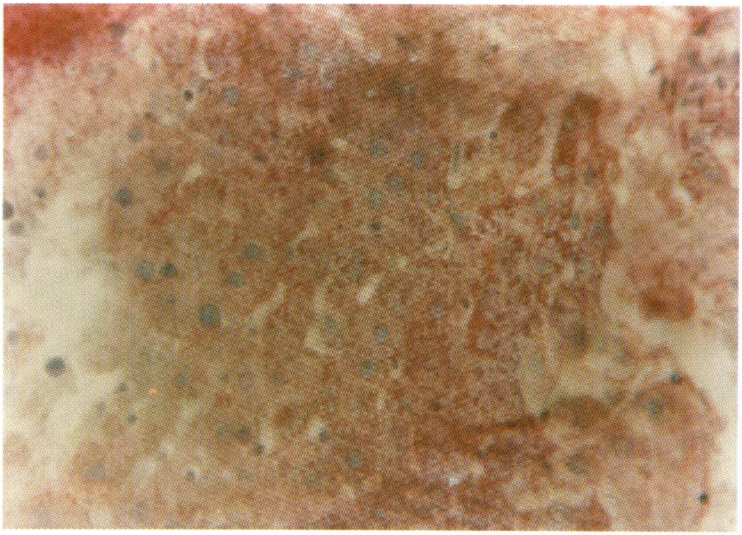

Fig. 4.9 : Thin section of DENA control rat liver (22 weeks after ip injection of DENA) showing dense rose-red coloured region indicating a much enhanced rate of periodic-acid-Schiff reaction (× 400).

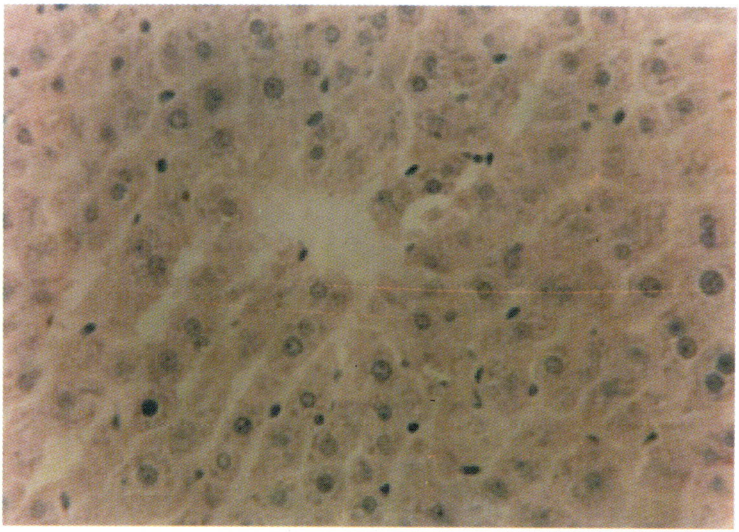

Fig. 4.10 : Section of rat liver (22 weeks after ip injection of DENA) plus concurrent administration of crude aqueous extract of *T. portulacastrum* (H and E × 400)

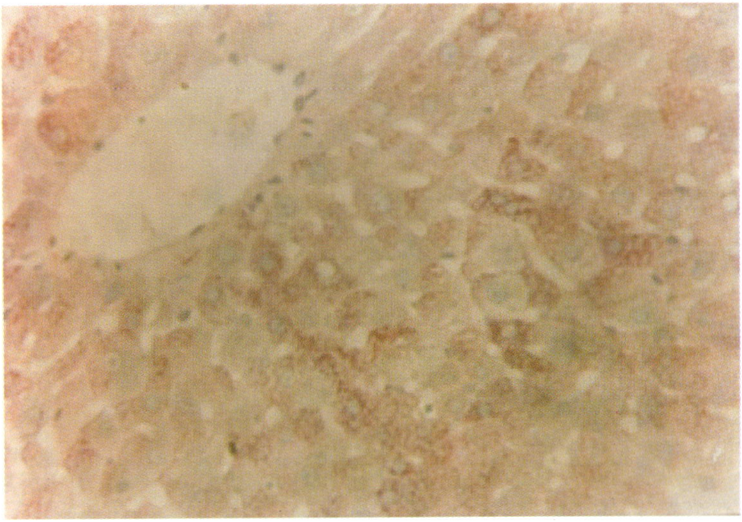

Fig. 4.11 : Thin section of rat liver (DENA + crude aqueous extract of *T. portulacastrum* indicating PAS positive zones (× 400).

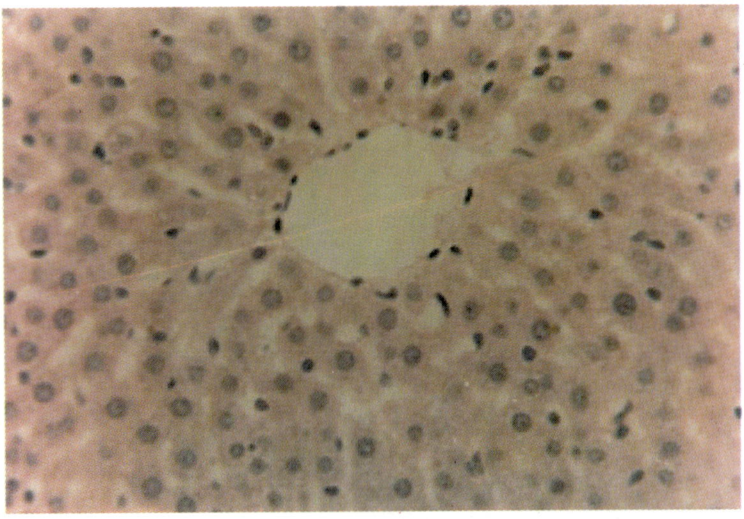

Fig. 4.12 : Section of rat liver (22 weeks after ip injection of DENA) plus concurrent administration of Ethanolic extract of *T. portulacastrum* (H and E × 400).

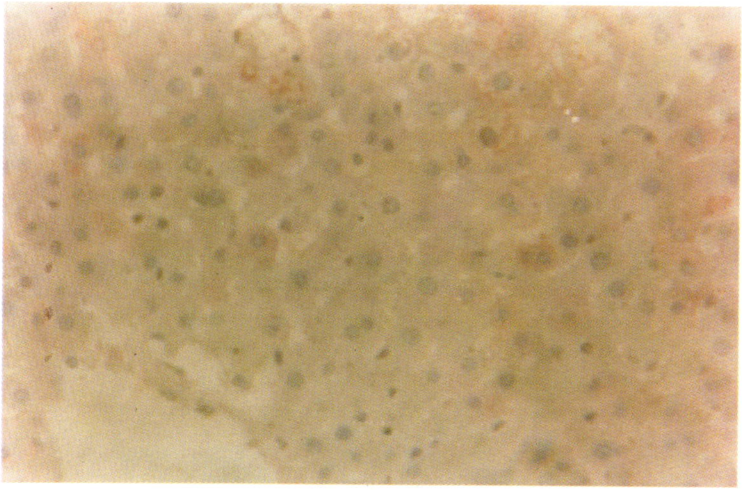

Fig. 4.13 : Thin section of rat liver (DENA + Ethanolic extract of *T. portulacastrum* revealing PAS positive areas (× 400).

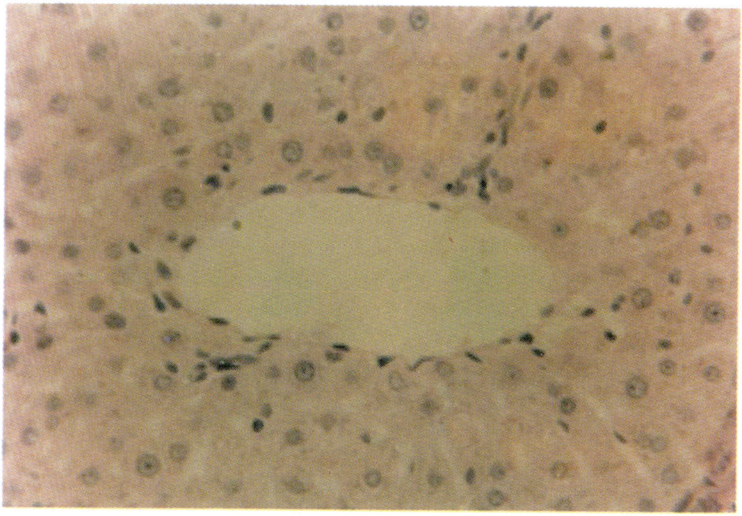

Fig. 4.14 : Section of rat liver indicating conspicuous recovery from hepatic carcinogenesis (ip injection of DENA + concurrent administration of $CHCl_3$ extract of *T. portulacastrum* (H and E × 400).

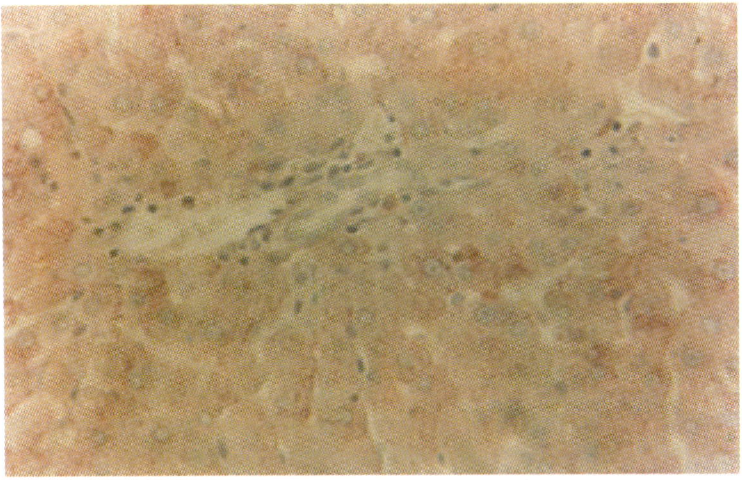

Fig. 4.15 : Thin section of rat liver (DENA + $CHCl_3$ extract of *T. portulacastrum* showing rose-red PAS positive zones almost similar to the normal untreated rat liver (× 400).

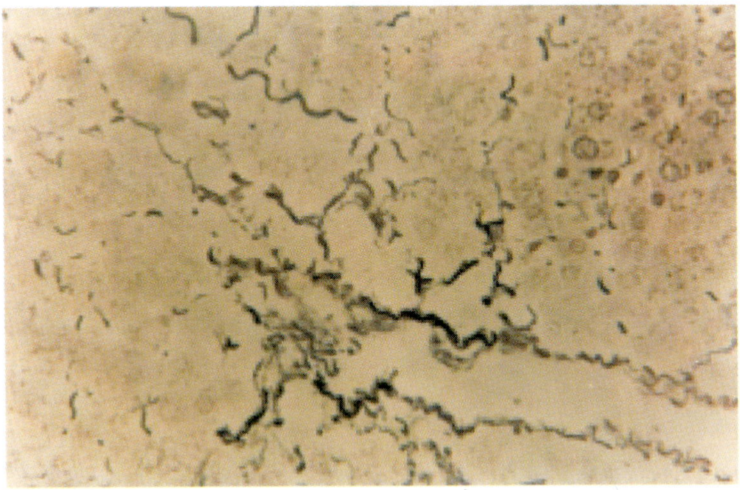

Fig. 4.16 : Arrangement of Reticulin fibres in DENA + $CHCl_3$ extract of *T. portulacastrum* treated group, showing almost normal arragement of the fibres.

Group C animals revealed near normal reticulin structure indicating that the crude aqueous extract of the plant was able to preserve the normal structure of reticulin against the onslaught of the necrogenic effect of DENA.

In Group D animals treated with the EtOH extract of *Trianthema portulacastrum*, only mild periportal increase of reticulin fibres were observed (figure not shown). The extract was effective in suppressing alteration of the gross fibrillar pattern of reticulin. Group E animals treated with the $CHCl_3$ fraction of the plant, displayed normal reticulin pattern compared to Group A animals. The marked anti-carcinogenic ability of the $CHCl_3$-extract of *T. portulacastrum* is further confirmed by the observation that the extract was a highly effective agent capable of suppressing apparent DENA-induced injuries as reflected by the normal orientation of reticulin fibres with no signs of fibrosis.

The retention of glycogen on fasting has been well established as one of the most important positive markers for pre-neoplastic hepaocytes (Farber, 1980). It is well known that both clear and eosinophillic cells, form multiple foci, during the pre-neoplastic phase. These lesions correspond to glycogen storage foci, during the pre-neoplastic phase and are characterized by an excessive storage of glycogen. Hepatocellular glycogenesis observed under the light microscope by the PAS reaction. A considerable accumulation of glycogen in cells of neoplastic nodules has also been demonstrated suggesting that the nodules originate from the foci storing glycogen in excess (Bannasch, 1978). Hepatocellular glycogenesis which has been described as the initial stage of neoplastic transformation of hepatocytes in experimental animals is a good cytochemical marker of the early steps in the development of human hepatic neoplasia (Bannasch, 1978).

Several reports are available regarding the appearance of hepatic tumours in adult patients, with inborn hepatic glycogenesis (Spycher and Gitzelmann, 1971; Howell *et al.*, 1976; Levine *et al.*, 1976).

The results of the present study reveal large number of glycogen storage cells in the foci and nodules 22 weeks following a single ip injection of DENA at a necrogenic dose of 200 mg/kg body weight in 0.9% NaCl (Ogawa *et al.*, 1980), which seems to be in line with the earlier report of the same hepatocarcinogen (Scherer *et al.*, 1972).

The observed DENA induced hepatocarcinogenesis exhibiting hepatocellular glycogenesis indicates considerable extent of pre-neoplasia also evident from the present histological evaluation.

Trianthema portulacastrum mediated reduction of glycogen storage in the altered hepatocytes, especially following a 22-week treatment, accumulates evidence regarding the ability of the extract in inhibiting the magniude of hepatic pre-neoplasia, and thereby ultimately incidence of liver cancer in rodents.

Since hepatocellular glycogenesis represents an early disregulation of carbohydrate metabolism during hepato-carcinogenesis, the plant extract mediated protection against DENA-induced metabolic disturbance, leading to glycogenesis, could be viewed to be an adaptation of the cellular enzymes which gradually redirects the carbohydrate metabolism towards glycolysis and pentose phosphate cycle (Nour-Eldeen *et al.*, 1985). The results of our present study establish a positively beneficial long term effect of the different fractions of *T. portulacastrum* in the experimental models under observation. The extract has a unique antitumorigenic potency which is amply confirmed by histopathological and histochemical observations of hepatic tissues of DENA treated rats.

Although the exact mechanism of action of the plant extract is still unknown the presence of the phenolic compounds such as Quercetin suggest that the extract suppresses caricinogenesis by its ability to modulate protein kinase enzyme (Mistry *et al.*, 1997). Alternatively it is possible that substances within the extract exert their effects by interaction with cellular signalling pathways. (Egan *et al.*, 1997).

5

Effect of the Chloroform Extract of *Trianthema portulacastrun* L. in Experimental Rat Hepatocarcinogenesis : An Ultrastructural Probe into the Changes

1. Introduction

Electron Microscopy, developed first in Germany by Ruska *et al.*, 1930, was extensively employed in molecular and cell biology, but clinical applications occurred more slowly. Now it is a widely accepted tool in the evaluation of undifferentiated neoplasms (Crook and Preiser, 1991).

Transmission Electron Microscopy (TEM)

Is analgous to the light microscope in many respects. Light source consists of a stream of electrons which are focussed on electromagnetic fields that act as lenses to create the final image. The specimen is embedded in plastic, sectioned and stained with heavy metal. As the electron passes through the specimen, some interaction with the heavy metal atoms takes place, thus scattering the electrons. The e^- beam is then focussed, magnified and projected onto a fluorescent screen. Areas of the sample which alter the passage of electrons, appear dark. Sample areas where no scatter occurrs appear white. Intermediate scattering produces a grey image.

Although most neoplasms can be correctly identified histologically, 5-10% seem to defy precise classification even after the application of routine special stains. Since 1960s EM is being routinely used to resolve these diagnostic dilemmas. In the rat hepatocarcinogenesis model employed in the study, drastic tissue level alterations brought about by a necrogenic dose of DENA have already been observed (Chapter IV of this book). Histologic profile of rat liver subjected to treatment with $CHCl_3$ extract of *Trianthema portulacastrum* immediately after DENA administration have also been observed. The remarkable chemopreventive efficacy of the $CHCl_3$ extract prompted as to look for the other changes, especially at the ultrastructural level, so that differences seen histologically become paralelled with findings at the ultrastructural platform. Histochemical studies may further provide supplemental information complementing light and ultrastructural features. In this study EM (TEM) was employed as a means of limiting a differential diagnosis and for confirming the ones suggested by other modalities (histology and histochemistry) (Table 5.1).

Table 5.1 : Electron Microscopy–Utility in Tumour Diagnosis

- Detects specific cell of origin, if specific diagnostic organelles are present eg. Melanomas.
- Narrows differential diagnosis down to a group of tumours.
- Confirms the impressions of other diagnostic modalities.
- Further refines a differential diagnosis arrived at by diagnostic techniques such as immunohistochemistry.
- Resolves conflicting impressions from different diagnostic approaches.
- Resolves an uncertain result from another usually newer diagnostic technique-specific ultra structural features in a tumour.

Usually specimens procured for diagnostic EM are solid tissues. Sometimes needle biopsies, fine needle aspirates, bone marrow aspirates, effussions and cerebrospinal fluids are used.

Chronic administration to rats-azodyes such as 3'-Me-DAB produces hepatic cell necrosis, oval cell or bile duct cell proliferation and nodular regenerative hyperplasia. At the level of fine structure, the changes induced in rat hepatocytes include proliferation of agranular endoplasmic reticulum, disorganization and loss of granular endoplasmic reticulum, glycogen depletion in rare cases, increase in the number of Lysosomes, lipid accumulation as well as alterations of the mitochondria, golgy apparatus and nucleus (Porter and Bruni, 1959; Svoboda *et al.*, 1964; 1968; Ketterer *et al.*, 1967; Flacks and Teh, 1975).

Single dose of hepatocarcinogens gives rise to hydropic degeneration, cellular swelling, or progressive vacuolation in rat hepatocytes (Flacks *et al.*, 1975). Large clear cytoplasmic areas containing unidentified small dark granules have also been reported (Arcasoy *et al.*, 1966; 1969).

Most neoplastic nodules represent a mixture of pre cancerous, definitively cancerous, and diverse intermediate cells as revealed from EM studies (Bannasch, 1976).

Marked differences in response to several hepatocarcinogens have been observed in the parenchymal cells of liver lobules. Centrilobular areas are more extensively affected than portal areas (Ketterer and Holt, 1967).

In view of the above, the present study was undertaken to observe 1) Major ultrastructural changes induced by a necrogenic dose of DENA–a potent hepatocarcinogen and 2) To observe the chemopreventive/anticarcinogenic potential of the $CHCl_3$ extract of *Trianthema portulacastrum* in reversing the pathological changes induced by DENA, following continuous treatment of the experimental animals with the extract at a dose of 100 mg/kg body weight once daily.

2. Materials and Methods

2.1 *Plant Material*

Dried overground parts of the plant *T. portulacastrum* L. were supplied by United Chemicals and Allied Products, Calcutta, India. The plant was authenticated by the Botanical Survey of India and a Voucher specimen no. (JUPharm/Biochem/SPO3) has been deposited in the same herbarium.

Extraction of the Plant Material

Airdried overground parts of *T. portulacastrum* L. were crushed in a waring blender and the fine pulverized material was subjected to exhaustive extraction in a Soxhlet's extractor with Petroluem ether (b.p. 60-80°C). The petroleum ether extract was discarded. The marc was then successively extracted with benzene, chloroform and acetone. Finally the residue was extracted with ethanol 95% w/v (Vohra *et al.*, 1983).

The liquid concentrate obtained in case of the chloroform extract was taken, and subjected to distillation in a distillating flask using a glass condenser. The distillation took about an hour. The extract was initially taken in a round bottomed flask placed within a heating mantle. The distillate was collected in another flat bottomed flask. The flask containing the extract and the flask containing the final distilled product were connected to a condenser, connected to a water source by rubber tubing. The heating mantle was fitted to an electric source. The distillate was eventually reduced to a solid residue by rotary vacuum evaporation below 45°C to yield 4.8% w/w of the chloroform extract of *Trianthema portulacastum*. It was stored at 4°C until use. Prior to anticarcinogenic evaluation, the chloroform fraction was suspended in deionized water. 0.2 ml of 0.05% Tween 80 was added to the sticky chloroform fraction in distilled water using a Potter-Elvehjhum homogeniser. Tween 80 was added as an emulsifying agent to enhance the solubility of the fraction in water.

Finally the sample solution was stirred in a magnetic stirrer using a teflon coated magnetic paddle, thereby ensuring uniform homogeneous sample of plant extract, ready for animal feeding.

Chemicals

"DENA" Sigma Chemical Co. St Louis U.S.A., Glutaraldehyde SRL, Ltd., Bombay India, Cacodylate buffer; Osmium tetroxide, EPON 812, Uranyl acetate, Lead citrate, Ethanol (E-Merk, Germany) were procured partly from C.S.I.R. centre for Biochemicals, and were partly provided by ALL INDIA INSTITUTE OF MEDICAL SCIENCES, E.M. Facility, Deptt. of Anatomy, New Delhi.

Animals

80 male sprague Dawley rats initially weighing 110-120 g, were obtained from Indian Institute of Chemical Biology, (C.S.I.R.), Calcutta, India. Animals were divided at random into 4 groups–Normal Control, Carcinogen Control, DENA+Chloroform extract treated Group and *Trianthema* $CHCl_3$ extract control group. Each group consisted of 20 rats, and the animals were housed 5 rats/cage in suspended wirebottomed galvanized cages, in rooms controlled for temperature (28±1°C) and relative humidity (60%±5) with 12 hour light/dark cycles. The animals had free access to standard pellet diet (Lipton India) and water adlibitum during the

entire experiment. Animals were acclamatized to the standard laboratory conditions for 10 days before actual experiments were started.

2.2 *Experimental Protocol*

All the experimental animals, except the normal control, and Trianthema $CHCl_3$ extract control group were administered a single ip injection of DENA as was done previously, following the method of Ogawa *et al.*, 1980. In the above experiment, Group A animals were Normal controls, Group B animals served as Carcinogen controls and Group C animals comprised the treatment group. Group D animals comprised of *Trianthema* $CHCl_3$ extract controls. Animals of Groups C and D were administered 100 mg/kg body wt, plant drug ($CHCl_3$ extract) of *Trianthema portulacastrum* once daily. Treatment with the extract was started one day after ip injection of DENA, providing the animals necessary time lag to recover from the initial stress produced by DENA-injection.

The experiment was continued for 22 weeks and at the end of the 22nd week, the animals were sacrificed under light ether aneasthesia, and samples were prepared for E.M. analysis.

2.3 *Treatment of Tissues for TEM*

A sample of the hepatic tissue was quickly dissected out and blotted dry and weighed in an electronic balance. About 0.30 g of tissue was scissored from the distal end of the median lobe of the livers of both control and treated animals. Hepatic tissue was then cut into tiny 1 mm^3 blocks (about the size of a pinhead) in ice-cold 4% w/v glutaraldehyde in 0.067M Cacodylate buffer pH 7.2 (Sabatini and Bensch, 1963; Epstein and Holt, 1963). Fixation was continued for 4 hours at 0-4°C. The fixed tissue was washed overnight by immersion in 0.1M sodium cacodylate in 0.25M sucrose before post fixation in phosphate buffered 1% osmiumtetroxide at 0-4°C for 2 hours. After dehydration, with graded strengths of aqueous alcohol, tissue fragments were embedded in EPON 812 according to the method of Luft (Luft, 1961).

For electron microscopy, ultrathin sections (100-500Å) exhibiting silver to light gold interference colours were cut on a

Sorvall MT-1 Porter-Blum ultramicrotome, using a diamond knife. Sections were then mounted on copper grids, double-stained with saturated uranyl acetate, in 50% ethanol and lead tartarate (Reynolds, 1963), prior to the examination in a Philips CM 10 electron microscope at an accelerating voltage of 60KV.

After TEM viewing for about 2 hours per sample, TEM photographs were taken at the E.M. Facility, Department of Anatomy, AIIMS, New Delhi.

3. Results

Electron microscopic investigations of neoplastic nodules during rat liver. Carcinogenesis have revealed that the proliferative lesions, display a rather heterogeneous cell population, comprised of a mixture of several types of altered hepatocytes. Nodules eventually progress into HCC's after a time lag (Bannasch, 1976). Hepatocytes composing nodules exhibit cytoplasmic changes, nuclear atypia and mitoses (Bannasch, 1976).

In the carcinogen control group i.e. Group B animals, E.M. micrograph 1 reveals drastic degenerative changes. Masses of dense glycogen particles are visible. These particles have taken a rosette appearance at certain places. Meandering cisternae of the smooth type endoplasmic reticulum is visible. The reticulum is agranal or poorly granal. Glycogen areas appear to be interwoven by a loose meshwork, that is mostly acidophillic, but with few basophillic dark spots. Kupfer cell hyperplasia is also prominent. e^- dense materials are present. EM micrograph 2 reveals an area of the nodule showing ruptured tissue. Dense glycogen granules are either clustered at places or are free separated from each other at long distances. EM micrograph 3 reveals liver parenchymal cells that have become very loose. Elongated processes are visible and the cytoplasm shows 2 types of vescicles, clear looking vescicles and dense vescicles. Other cytoplasmic structures are barely discerable. Hepatocytes possess a single large nucleus with nucleolus. Nucleus is a typical with irregular outline. Nucleolar structure cannot be detailed from the figure. It is lumpy in appearance. Heterochromatin is considerably reduced in quantity. Cytoplasmic organelles seem to be absent.

The change is quite drastic with enormous changes in cytological details and structure. There is evidence for presence of

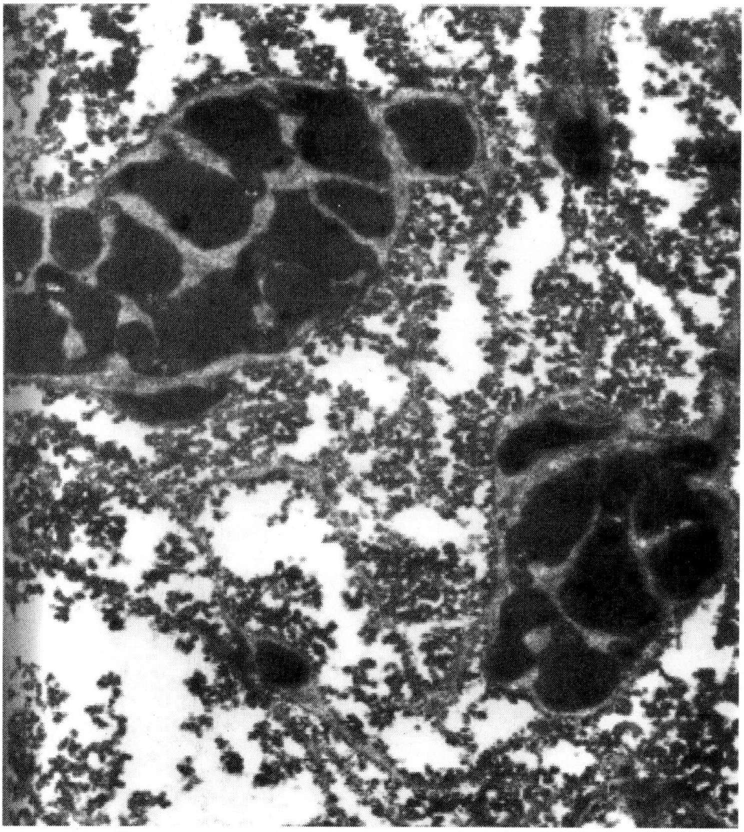

Micrograph 1
F × 3400
S × 10,500

1-2 mitochondria in the hepatocytes, when the normal count is 2000 EM micrograph 4 shows very loose arrangement of cells. Cytoplasm appears to be highly vacuolated, loose attachment sites are quite prominent., indicating absence of desmosomes. EM micrographs 5 and 6 reveal vacuolated cytoplasm, ruptured tissue areas, dense clusters of glycogen forming a meshwork. An unindentified greyish body, much elongated in shape seems to be occupying the vacuoles.

A marked change in the fine structural organization of the rat hepatocyte was therefore apparent. The most conspicuous and

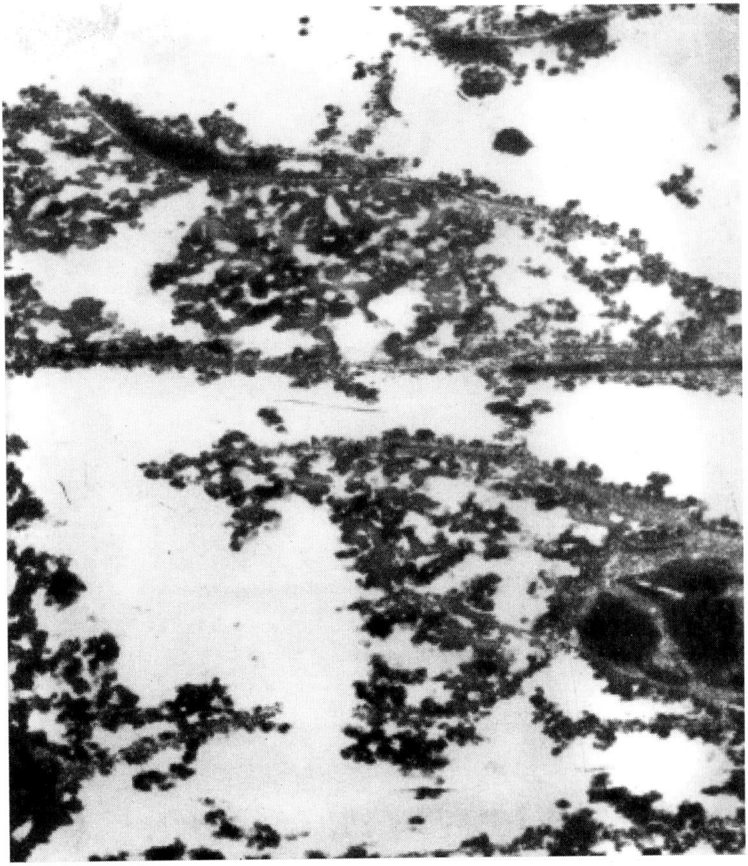

Micrograph 2
F × 3400
S × 10,500

consistent alteration was the peripheral displacement of cytoplasmic organelles, by the grossly enlarged glycogen areas. In the more severely affected cells, nuclei were irregular with kinky outline, interconnection between the cells was loose, and moderately increased quantities of agranular endoplasmic reticulum were observed.

Group A animals (normal Controls), Group D (*Trianthema* $CHCl_3$ extract controls) (figures not shown) displayed normal

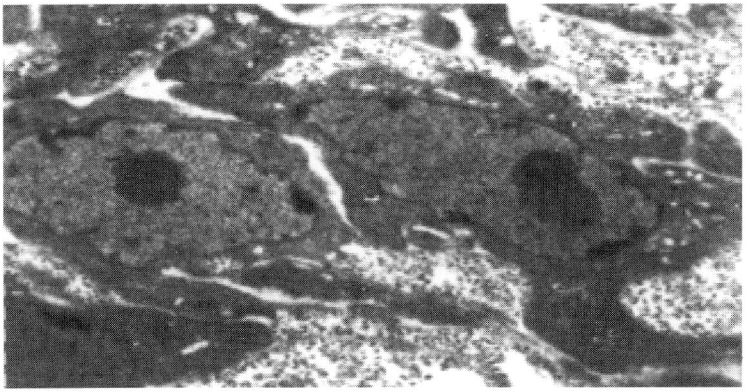

Micrograph 3
F × 4600 S × 1350

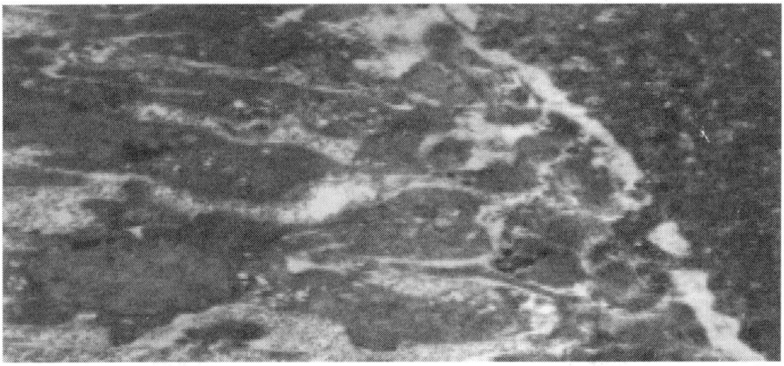

Micrograph 4
F × 790 S × 2650

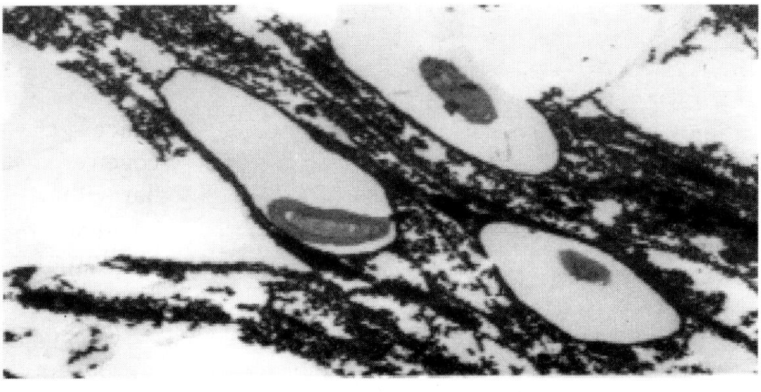

Micrograph 5
F × 870 S × 2600

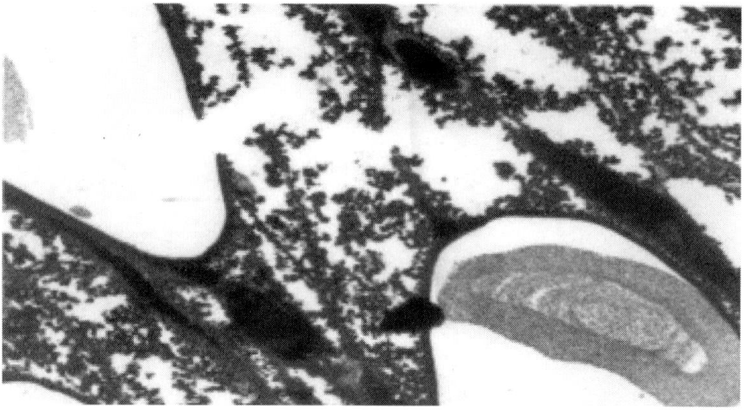

Micrograph 6
F × 790
S × 2650

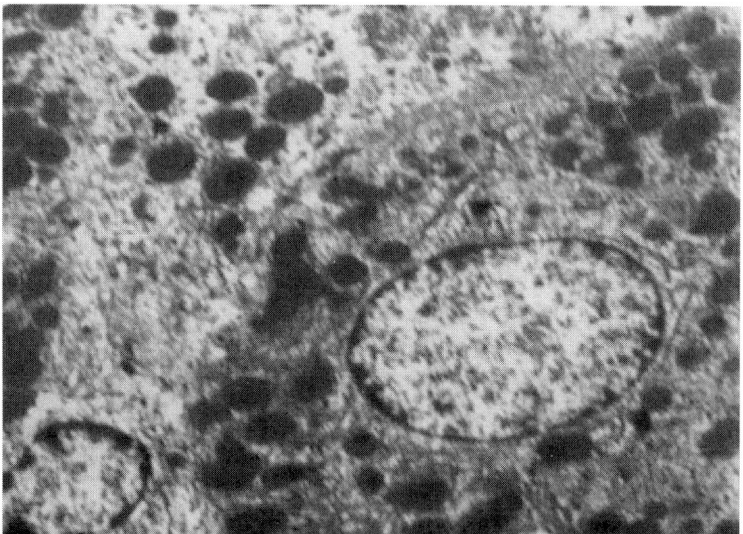

Micrograph 7
F × 1950
S × 5800

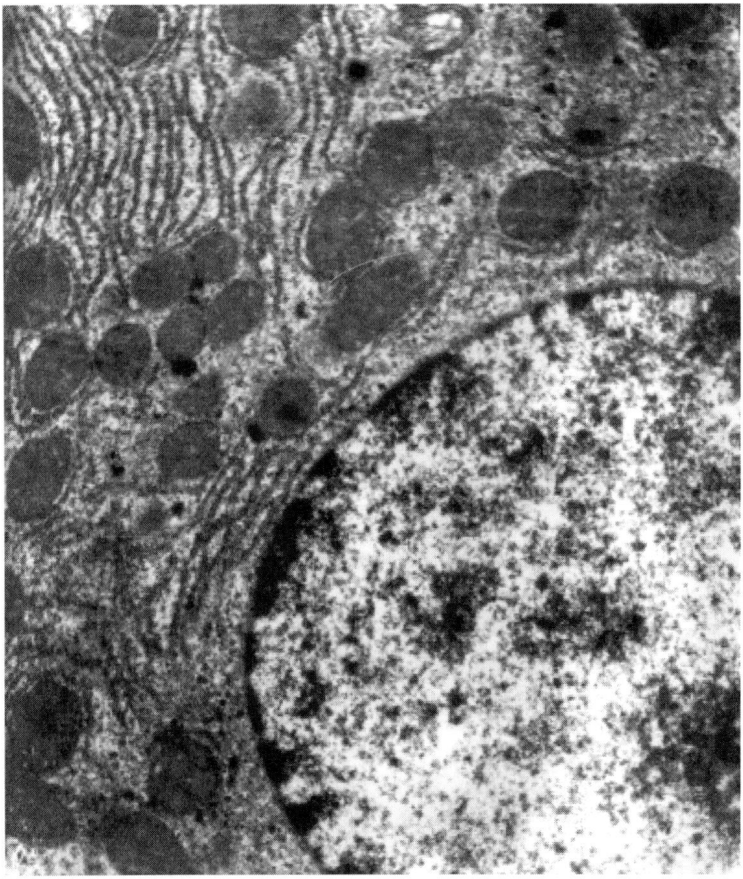

Micrograph 8
F × 3400
S × 10,500

features of hepatocytes with plenty of rough surfaced E.R. with characteristic stacks of flattened cisternae studded with ribosomes. Free polysomes and free ribosomes were located at intercisternal spaces. Smooth E.R. was found in association with golgy apparatus, and also in glycogen containing regions. No loosening of cells was discernable from the samples. Golgy bodies showed typical forming and maturing areas in the form of zones.

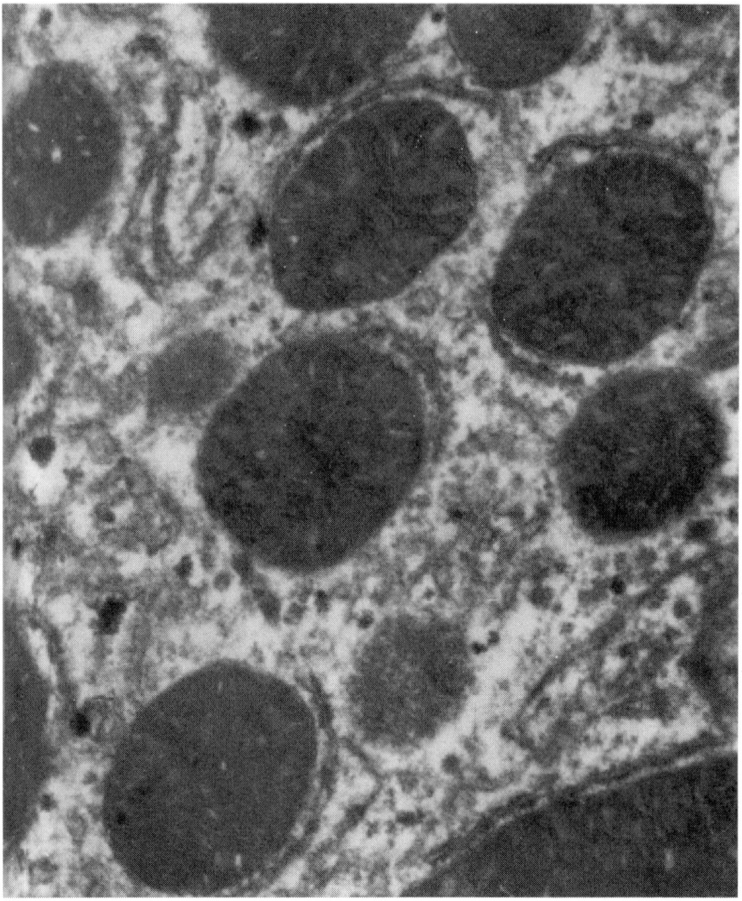

Micrograph 9
F × 8100
S × 2500

Group C animals were DENA injected and treated with chloroform extract of *Trianthema portulacastrum.* EM micrograph 7 shows only slight loosening of neighbouring hepatocytes. The extreme loosening found in Group B animals seems to be largely overcome in Group C animals supplemented with *Trianthema portulacastrum* in their diet. The loose spaces are filled with fibro-granular substances. The nucleus looked normal, but was devoid of nucleolus. EM micrograph 9 shows the arrangement and

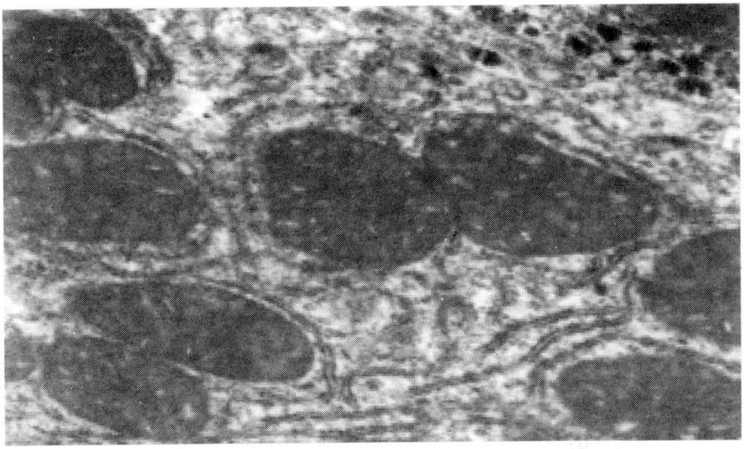

Micrograph 10
F × 8400
S × 2500

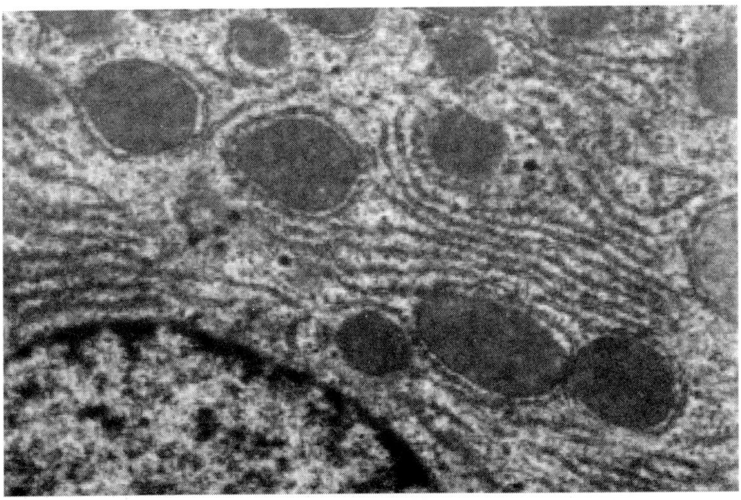

Micrograph 11
F × 4600
S × 13,500

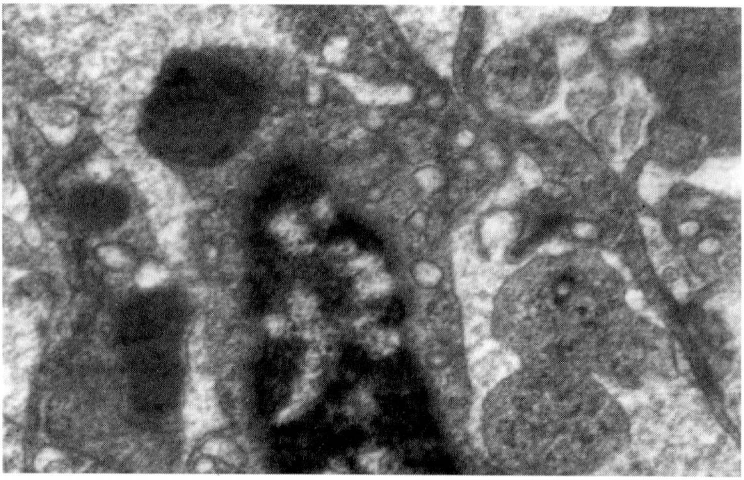

Micrograph 12
F × 3400
S × 10,500

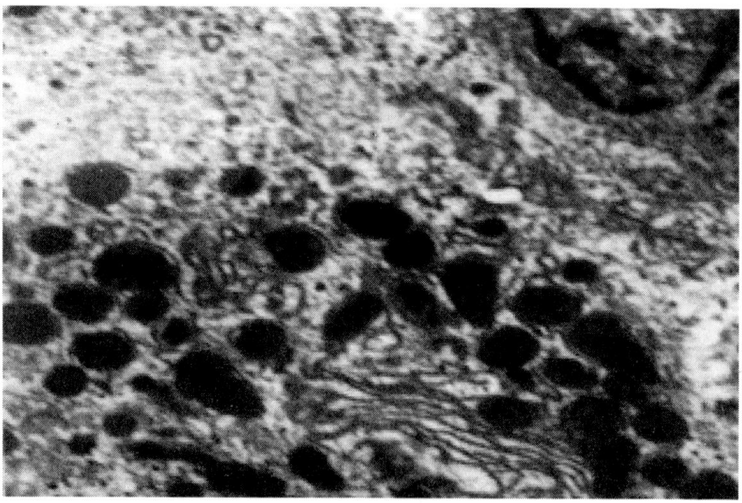

Micrograph 13
F × 1550
S × 7900

distribution of the mitochondria that appear to be quite normal. The matrices of the mitochondria seem to reveal varying amount of electron densities. Matrices are of 3 types, -low density, intermediate density and high density types. EM micrograph 8 shows the nucleus with deeply stained heterochromatic zones, in plentiful quantity, much like that in a normal hepatocyte. Peroxisomes appear to be present in average numbers. In certain places, peroxisomes are plenty. The core of the peroxisomes are without poly-microtubules. In the normal counterpart, peroxisomes contain a central crystalline core of urate oxidase. Urate oxidase is present in most of the peroxisomes of Group C animals.

EM micrograph 10 shows E.R. of rough type. E.R. is not uniformly developed in all the cells.

E.M. micrograph 11 reveals that in some of the cavities of the ER of the rough type a series of pin head like structures are visible. EM 12 shows kupfer cells found in average numbers in the cells, with no signs of hyperplasia. In such cells cytoplasm shows evidence of active pinocytosis.

From EM micrograph 13 it is seen that golgy apparatus are found in normal numbers as in Group A animals. In some cells, golgy regions show no differentiation into forming and maturing zones. Glycogen appears to be present in all the cells as is expected in normal cells.

On the whole, it is seen that *Trianthema portulacastrum* treatment to DENA injected animals brought about remarkable recovery to the nearly normal hepatocyte structure with cytological and karyological features closely approaching the normal controls.

Trianthema portulacastrum L., ($CHCl_3$ extract), thus displayed once again a strong anti-carcinogenic potential in reversing the necrogenic effects of the hepatocarcinogen, at last that mediated by DENA.

4. Discussion

Neoplastic nodules contain four types of altered hepatocytes– clear cells which store excess glycogen; which appear in the form of alpha and Beta particles (Drochmans *et al.*, 1972) acidiophillic cells presenting ground glass appearance, vacuolated cells containing lipid droplets and glycogen and basophillic cells devoid of glycogen (Bannasch, 1976; Karasaki *et al.*, 1969).

Hepatocarcinogens such as 3'- Me DAB has been reported to induce a marked change in the fine structural organization of the rat hepatocyte (Flacks *et al.*, 1975).

One of the earliest effects on the rat liver of a number of hepatotoxins and carcinogens is to produce alterations in the rough surfaced ER of parenchymal cells (Ketterer *et al.*, 1967). A single dose of DMNA, caused break down of the characteristic lamellar organization of the reticulum and a marked increase in the number of free ribosomes (Emmelot and Benedetti, 1961). CCl_4, aflatoxin and other carcinogens bring about dilation and vesciculation of the cisternae, of ER, dispersal of ribosomes and loss of ordered arrays followed by an accumulation of smooth surfaced membranes (Smuckler *et al.*, 1969). The ER has attracted considerable attention because of its role in chemical carcinogenesis in the liver. This is because it converts non-carcinogenic substances into metabolites implicated in carcinogenesis (Miller and Miller, 1967; Arcasoy *et al.*, 1967).

The classic liver lobule is a hexagon with portal triads at each corner. Hepatocytes are separated by blood sinusoids. The hepatocyte possess three surfaces. The apical surface lines a small lumen between adjacent cells defined by junctional complexes. Lateral surfaces contain junctions that define cell polarity and bind hepatocytes together (desmosomes) and provide communication between gap junctions. The basal surface is directly adjacent to the sinusoidal epithelium.

In the study, animals belonging to Group A (normal untreated controls) exhibited features of normal hepatocytes. The ER (rough type) had closely attached ribosomes, indicating active protein synthesis. The mitochondria were plenty indicating active cell respiation. Golgy bodies were being formed in series from the region of formation to the region of maturation. Glycogen content was normal, and cells were tightly cemented together with no loosening noticeable in any of the preperations. Group B animals (carcinogen controls) however revealed marked ultrastructural changes under the necrogenic influence of DENA. Drastic degenerative changes were observed in the nodules. Glycogen masses were aggregated presenting a rosette appearance. Granular

ER was much reduced and the ER of the smooth type prevailed in all the specimens observed in the different grids. Kupfer cells inhabiting the liver sinusoids, displayed hyperplasia, the nucleus was a typical with irregular outline. Heterochromatin was considerally reduced. A very loose arrangement of cells was a notable feature of the cells, clearly indicating the absence of desmosomes.

By contrast Group C animals, subjected to *Trianthema portulacastrum* treatment presented a different picture altogether. Hepatocytes had recovered considerably and closely resembled that of the normal untreated controls. The loosening of cells was much arrested and only feeble loosening between the cells were noted. Cytoplasmic features were quite normal in that mitochondia had increased in number, peroxisomal distribution was normal and golgy bodies were found in average counts. The nuclear margin was smooth with ample heterochromatin, observed as darkly stained areas on the nucleus in the EM micrographs.

The anticarcinogenic potential of the $CHCl_3$ extract of *T. portulacastrum* is thus confirmed and established from EM studies. The extract has proved remarkable in suppressing and/ or arresting the degenerative changes, brought about by DENA, a potent hepatocarcinogen. It has successfully prevented nodular formation, thereby preventing cytologic and karyologic damages, seen in typical neoplastic nodules, produced by a single i.p. injection of DENA.

The findings at the ultrastructural level have matched with the findings at the histological level, and cytochemical level.

Glycogen rich e^- dense granules, visible in the nodules in EM micrographs are paralelled by the deep rose-red areas of periodic acid schiff reaction, indicated by the PAS positive zones in the histochemical studies of the hyperplastic nodules. Further studies are underaway to isolate and or to identify the components which are responsbile for repairing the cellular damage of the subcellular particles.

6

Suppression of Chromosomal Aberrations by the Chloroform Extract of *Trianthema portulacastrum* L in Experimental Hepatic Tumorigenesis

1. Introduction

Neoplasia is characterized by deregulated cell proliferation and phenotypic abnormalities, that confer properties of invasion and metastasis (Masahiro *et al.*, 1996). Activation of telomerase in the hyperplastic nodules and HCC's is required to achieve immortality and proceed to the malignant state. (Toshifumi *et al.*, 1996).

Cancer has been referred to as a genetic disturbance, which itself has a genetics (German, 1985). At the cellular level, cancer can be considered a genetic disturbance as critical events in tumorigenesis include alterations in DNA. (Testa *et al.*, 1991).

In most tumours there are genomic alterations, that are visible at the light microscope level as karyotypic changes. At least two types of genes with relevance to cancer have been identified. Oncogenes act in a dominant fashion, directly transforming certain target cells. Tumour suppressor genes or anti-oncogenes are recessive at the cancer genes, which require that loci of both chromosomal homologues become inactivated before a tumour can occur. There is a vast amount of cytogenetic evidence, both circumstantial and direct implicating cancer chromosome abnormalities as somatic cell mutations critical in tumorigenesis (Heim and Mitelman 1987).

Investigations into Karyotypic abnormalities in experimental animals demands an arrest of the dividing neoplastic cells in metaphase or late prophase, with acceptable spreading, fixation of chromosomes and high quality banding of chromosomes prior to microscopic examination.

DENA is potent liver carcinogen, in all mammalian species tested (IARC Monographs, 1972). It is potent inducer of chromosome aberrations and sister chromatid exchanges (SCE's) in cultured mammalian cells, in the presence of rat liver microsomal system (Natarajan *et al.*, 1976; Matsuoka *et al.*, 1979; Horiuchi *et al.*, 1984).

The participation of chromosomal abnormalities in tumour inhibition and promotion, is well documented as suggested by the association of specific chromosomal rearrangements with particular cancers (Gilbert, 1983). Further Chromosomes, that are responsible for deviation of stem-line karyotypes are in reality those that carry genes, with specific significance for malignant development. (Levan *et al.*, 1977). Cellular DNA is involved in bringing about changes in chromosomal patterns. Observations at the level of chromosomes, is a crude method to elucidate changes in the cellular DNA, yet findings of consistent chromosomal patterns in neoplasia have been found to be meaningful. (Rowley *et al.*, 1977; Rowley, 1980). Chromosomal aberrations (CA's) are important somatic mutations, and are involved in the origin, progression and diversification of certain cancer types. (Nowell, 1976; Land *et al.*, 1983). However it is difficult to characterize aberrations crucial for initiation and early stages of tumour development. In view of the acknowledged importance of CA as a hall mark of the stage of progression in multistage carcinogenesis, the present study was undertaken to get an insight into the critical CAs involved in early stages of hepatic neoplasia by DENA, and its possible alteration by *Trianthema Portulacastrum*.

Karyotypic analysis of the stages of rat hepatocarcinogenesis has been able to identify specific chromosomal loci involved in the development and progression of neoplasms (Rowley, 1980; Mitelman *et al.*, 1990). In addition karyotypic analysis has permitted identification and characterization of tumour suppressor gene loci. The WB rat liver epithelial cell line was developed from a normal F 344 rat liver (Tsao *et al.*, 1984). This cell line and its derivatives have proved useful in the characterization of rat liver carinogenesis (Tsao *et al.*, 1985; Lee *et al.*, 1989; 1991).

Coleman *et al.*, (1995) have used several variants of this cell line to demonstrate the importance of tumour suppressor locus on rat chromosome 3 and have concluded that the region corresponding to human 11 p 12 is important in the genesis or early progression of rat liver epithelial cells. Studies in this line have indicated that several loci are of potential importance in the genesis of HCC in rats and they are located within the region of chromosome 1 that gets frequently altered in models of rat liver cancer. (Wolman *et al.*, 1973; Kovi *et al.*, 1983; Sargent *et al.*, 1992).

These findings and several others have shown that the malignant phenotype arises as a result of consistent chromosomal aberrations (Solomon *et al.*, 1991). In view of the above, the chemopreventive efficacy of the extract ($CHCl_3$ extract of *Trianthema Portulacastrum*) in arresting hepatocarcinogenesis of rodents in relation to the genetic parameters, was studied.

2. Materials and Methods

2.1 *Plant Material*

Pulverized plant material of *T. portulacastrum* L. were used to make chloroform extract of the plant, by the same procedure followed in the earlier chapter (Chapter 5).

2.2 *Animals*

80 male sprague-Dawley rats weighing 110-120g were obtained from Indian Institute of Chemical Biology, C.S.I.R, India. The animals were maintained on purified basal diet (lipton India), Containing 25% protein and water adlibitum, until their bodyweights reached 130-150g range. They were then divided at random into various experimental and control groups. Group A animals (20 in number) served as the normal untreated controls. Group B animals (20 in number were the carcinogen controls). Group C animals comprised the treatment Group. Group D animals served as *Trianthema* controls and received only the extract and no DENA. All animals of groups B and C were administered a single ip injection of DENA following the method

of Ogawa *et al.*, (1980) at a dose of 200 mg/kg body weight in 0.9% NaCl solution.

Group C animals were fed $CHCl_3$ extract of *Trianthema Portulacastrum* at a dose of 100 mgs/kg body weight once daily. This was a long term experiment, and was continued for 48 weeks. Towards the end of the 48th week, animals were fasted, and on the 48th week animals were sacrificed and peripheral blood collected for preparation of Chromosome slides, G-banding and Karyotype study.

2.3 *Analysis of Chromosomes from Peripheral Blood*

Peripheral blood culture technique is now almost Universally practised and its use extends to practically all vertebrates (Sharma and Sharma 1980). The method is based on the finding that under the influence of phytohaemagglutinin (PHA) the mitogenic agent of red kidney beans. *Phaseolus Vulgaris, P. Communis*, the lymphocytes in the peripheral blood participate in a "blastoid reaction" and get morphologically transformed into a blast like cell that divides in culture. In this study the macromethod for short-term tissue culture of Rat-peripheral blood was employed (Priest *et al.*, 1969).

Chemicals

Phytohaemagglutinin M type (DIFCO Code 0528), Calf serum, Dulbecco and Voght's medium, heparin, Colchicine, CIBA, India, Trypsin (DIFCO) and Giemsa stain were procured from diverse authentic sources.

2.4 *Experimental Protocol for Peripherial Blood Culture (Modification of that followed for humans)*

- 2 ml syringe taken, and running blood about 0.5 ml, drawn up in the syringe. (Done twice to make the blood volume upto 1.0 ml)
- Quickly added to sterilized tubes, containing 0.5 ml heparin.
- R.B.C's. permitted to settle out.
- Plasma carefully aspirated with pasteur pipette, leaving aside R.B.C.

- Leucocyte Count made with the Plasma in haemocytometer. (Total cell count should be at least 2×10^6/ml).
- Added 1ml plasma to culture medium in 2-0Z culture container.
- Added 0.2 ml Phytohaemagglutin M type well shaken and incubated at 37°C.
- Put into culture medium (Dulbecco and Voght's medium) enriched with 15% foetal calf serum and Phenol red indicator. pH maintained at 7.4.
- Incubated for 72 hours, with intermittent shaking.

The major steps in the preparation of metaphase plates for karyotype study from leucocyte culture, involve metaphase arrest, hypotonic treatment, fixation, preparation, staining.

2.5 *Preparation of Chromosomes from Peripheral Blood*

- After 72 hrs. incubation added sterile colchicine to a final concentration of 0.5 μg/ml.
- Incubation with colchicine continued upto 5 hours.
- Poured medium into centrifuge tubes, centrifuged at 800 rpm for 8 minutes.
- Supernatant poured off. Added several ml PBS. Cells suspended gently, by pushing out with Pasteur pipette.
- Recentrifuged as before.
- Removed supernatant, leaving only 0.5 ml. filled to 2ml mark with distilled water.
- Cells suspended gently as before.
- Incubated at 37°C for 10 minutes, shaken gently, centrifuged as before.
- Supernatant aspirated, as close to the top of the button as possible.
- Added 2 ml (1:3) acetic methanol (fixative) without disturbing button of cells.
- Made to stand at room temperature for 30 minutes.
- Cells resuspended by pushing out with Pasteur pipette.

- Centrifuged as before, supernatant, fully aspirated.
- Added 0.2 ml 45% acetic acid (to increase nuclear and chromosome spread). Dense cell suspension thus prepared.
- Added less for small button.
- Pre-cleaned chilled, dry, grease free slides kept ready.
- Moderately heavy cell suspension made to drop on the slides. Drop allowed to fall from a height of several inches down into the slide. Slide held at 60-90º angle and drop of cell suspension, allowed to run down the slide quickly. Excess liquid removed with blotting paper.
- Slides allowed to dry completely in slanted position prior to staining.

2.6 *Giemsa or G-Banding*

Giemsa is a complex mixture of thiazine dyes and eosin. Out of these methylene blue, Azure A, B and C give good banding. Thiazine dyes are strongly metachromatic and their absorption spectra and extinction coefficients change with increase in dye concentration or on binding to positively charged chromotypes (Comings, 1975). Strong banding is favoured by presence in the stain, high concentrations of methylene violet and its immediate homologues. Heated giemsa solution produces more consistent band on mammalian chromosomes (Vass and Sellyei, 1972; 1973). During G-banding macromolecules like DNA and proteins seem to be lost and leads to an uneven distribution of chromatin (Matsui and Sasaki 1975).

The amount of macromolecule residual after G-banding approximates two morphological bands. Residual proteins in G-bands are small molecules containing many S-S bands and possibly represent more stabilized DNA. G-positive bands thus represent relatively thermostable chromatins, consisting of smaller non-histone protein molecules (Sharma and Sharma, 1980). G-bands reveal intercalary bands and helps to identify each chromosome and any structural change that might have occurred. Some chemical carcinogens at concentrations producing transformation in vitro, can produce G-bands in human and hamster chromosomes after 24 hours treatment, possibly due to non-specific toxicity (Di Paolo and Popescu, 1974). Similar bands were observed in mouse bone narrow preparations of chromosomes, after injections in vivo of DNA-alkylating agents (Kitchin and Louden Slager, 1976).

In this experimental study, the necrogenic effect of DENA in producing characteristic bands, plus the protective effect of the extract were assessed in the light of G-banding and Karyotype analysis of the samples. The experimental set up, was a long term, experiment designed to get a clear picture from the haematological chromosome preparations, because reflections of the aberrations become apparent in the blood only after a period of 48 weeks, more precisely, the effect of DENA is seen not until this time gap, and only after a long time span, a stable karyotype is obtained.

Unlike "Q" and "C" bands, G-bands do not require any denaturation, renaturation (Drets and Shaw, 1971; Schendl, 1973; Hansen and Melander, 1974). G-banding is obtained by treatments in a variety of chemicals like standard saline NaOH/HCl before incubation. NaOH, trypsin etc. (Sea Bright, 1972; Sumner *et al.*, 1973; Hecht *et al.*, 1974) and sometimes even by mere heating (Lomholt and Mohr 1971). Treatment for 10 minutes in collagenase (50 μg/ml) solution in Ca^{++} and Mg^{++} free Hank's solution (pH 6.5) of mitotic slides from leucocyte cultures, followed by Giemsa staining gives G-bands (Trusler, 1975).

2.7 Procedure for G-Banding of Chromosomes from fresh airdried preparations of leucocytes

Chromosomes obtained from leucocytes were banded according to the method of Yunis and Sanchez, 1975.

- Kept slides in absolute methanol for 10 minutes.
- Slides allowed to airdry.
- Next stained with Giemsa 1/80 solution in 0.13 M phosphate buffer at pH 6.7.
- Allowed to remain for 30 minutes.
- Excess stain washed under running tap water, air dried.
- Observed under Adcon microscope for metaphase plates.

Well spread, well fixed, well banded plates were photographed.

2.8 *Scoring of C.A. data*

The slides were coded to avoid observer bias. The coded slides were blind scored. Metaphase plates showing one or more types of CA's were scored from at least 10 well spread metaphase plate/rat (i.e., 200 metaphase plates/Group) and the frequency of CA was expressed as the percentage of total aberrant metaphase plates. Aberrations were classed into 3 major groups according to published criteria (Sarkar *et al.*, 1994b). Group I comprised of structural aberrations and included gaps, breaks, deletions, fragments, centric fusions, rings, translocations (i.e., direct effect on Chromosomes). Group II comprised of numerical aberrations, represented by polyploidy and aneuploidy (i.e., direct effect on spindle apparatus). Group III consisted of physiological aberrations and included such aberrations as stickiness, Pycnosis, C-mitotic effect and pulverization (lethal effects).

3. Results and Discussion

A single ip injection of DENA administered to Group "B" animals resulted in an enhanced percentage of aberrant metaphase plates, as revealed from the chromosomes obtained from blood culture (Table 1). As menioned earlier, chromosomes from the blood of experimental animals were isolated after 48 weeks, because stable karyotypes are obtained only after a time lag. Immediate effect of DENA. With respect to the genetic parameters, can however be obtained from the liver, by partial hepatectomy (Horiuchi *et al.*, 1984) and DENA has been reported to cause Karyotypic alterations in the liver cells of rats (Grover and Fischer, 1971; Prince Hitachi *et al.*, 1974).

DENA has proved to be an effective inducer of micronuclei in adult rat liver cells (Tates *et al.*, 1980) or in mouse foetal liver derived erythroid cells (Cole *et al.*, 1982). The genotoxic effect of DENA was thus elaborated in this study.

From this long-term experimental study, it was observed that DENA mostly produced structural aberrations resulting in a direct damaging effect on chromosomes. Structural aberrations mostly resulted from breakage and rearrangement of whole chromosomes into abnormal forms. Both stable and unstable aberrations were induced by DENA. In the above experiment, stable aberrations that were observed included translocations,

Table 6.1 : Effect of *T. portulacastrum* on the frequency distribution of CA's of rat leucocytes in DENA-induced rat hepatocarcinogenesis.

Groups	No. of rats/ group	No. of meta-phase plates/ rat and total No. of plates		Structural CA's				Numerical CA's		Physiological CA's		Total CA		Protection
		No. of plates/ rats	No. of plates/ group	Individual type i.e. chromatid break, gap fragment		Exchange type centric fusions rings, trans-locations		Aneuploidy and polyploidy		Erosion, pulverisation stickyness				
				No.	%	No.	%	No.	%	No.	%	No.	%	%
A	20	10	200	0	0	0	0	0	0	1	0	1	0.5% ±0.2	
B	20	10	200	92	46%	68	34%	30	15%	10	5%	200	100% ±4.67[a]	
C	20	10	200	24	12%	18	9%	6	3%	4	2%	52	26% ±4.30[b]	74%
D	20	10	200	0	0	0	0	0	0	0	0	1	0.5 ±0.2	

[a]$P < 0.001$ compared to group A

[b] $P < 0.001$ compared to group B

% protection is expressed against group 'B'.

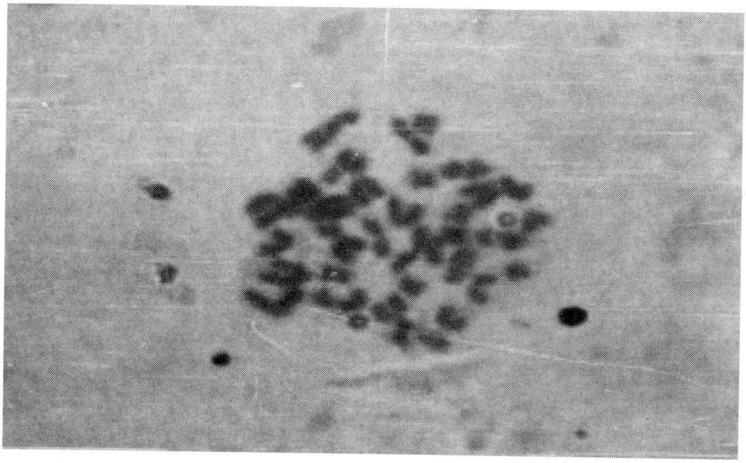

Fig. 6.1 : Metaphase plate from DENA-control rat showing translocation at two sites and centric fusion at a third site.

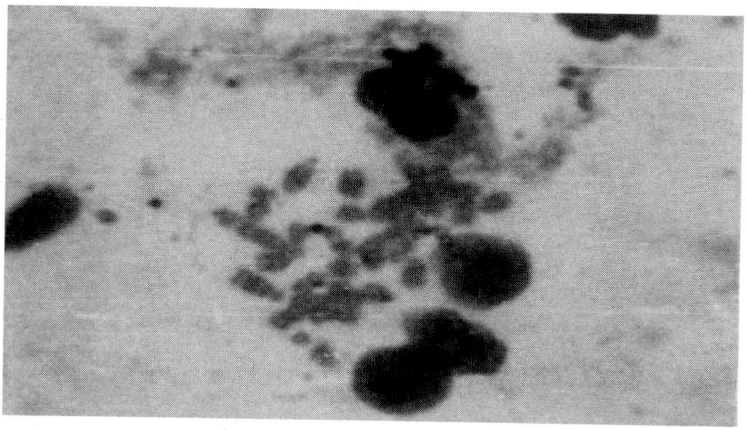

Fig. 6.2 : Metaphase plate from DENA-control rat showing region of chromatid gap

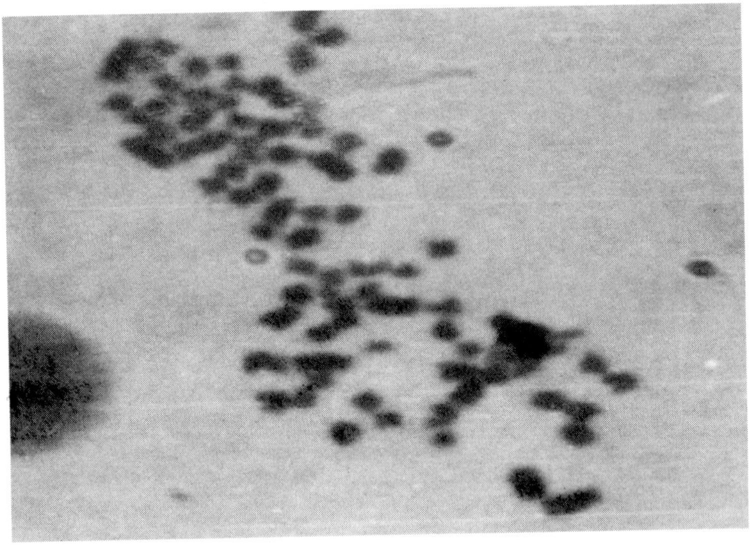

Fig. 6.3 : Aberrant metaphase plate from DENA-control rat showing an increase in the ploidy level.

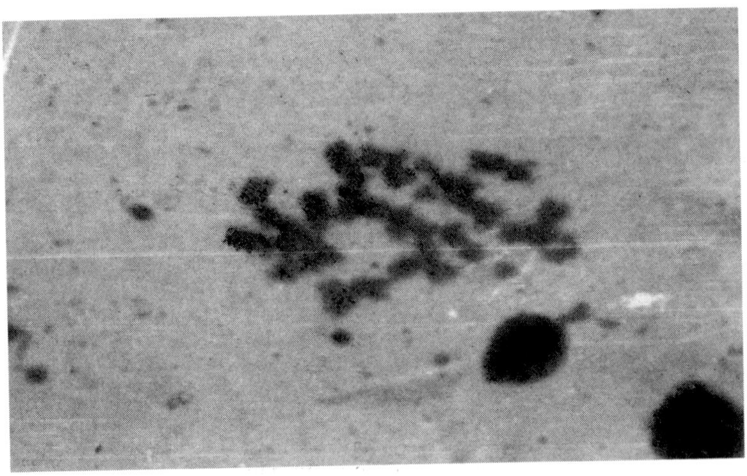

Fig. 6.4 : Aberrant metaphase plate from DENA-control rat, indicating the sticky nature of chromosomes.

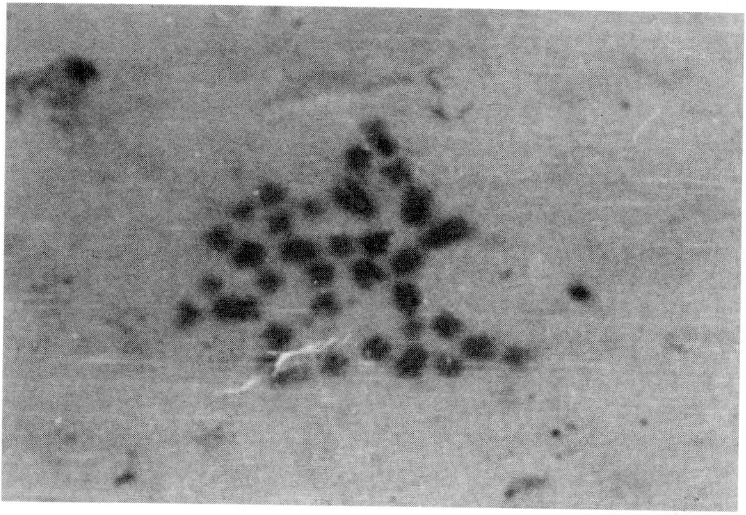

Fig. 6.5 : Well spread metaphase plate from DENA + $CHCl_3$ extract of *T. portulacastrum* treated group, displaying no observable aberration.

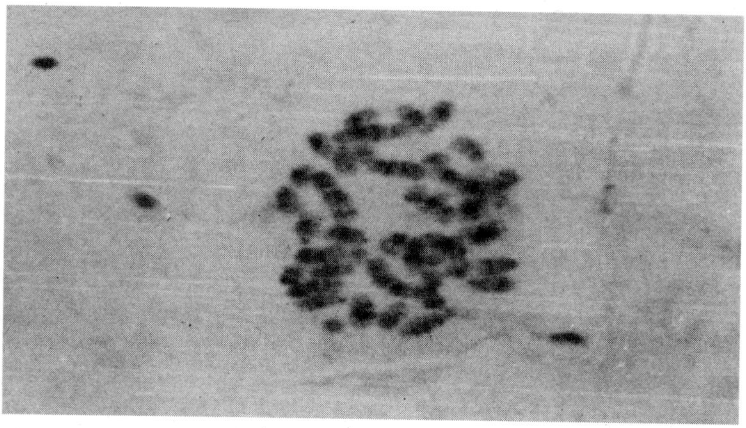

Fig. 6.6 : G-banded chromosomes of DENA control group, showing numerous breakage areas.

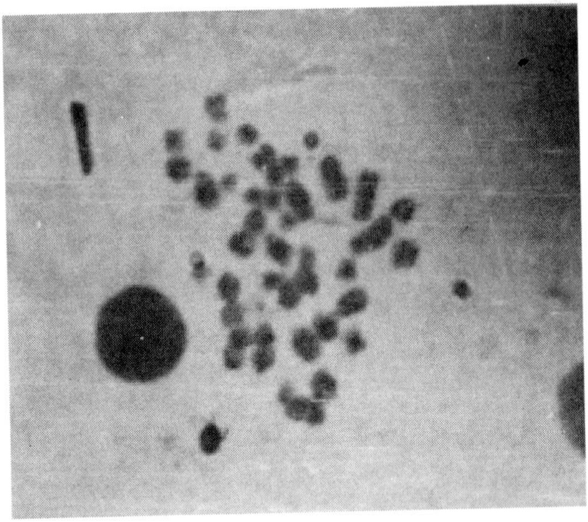

Fig. 6.7 : G-banded chromosomes from the treatment group (DENA + $CHCl_3$ extract of *T. portulacastrum*), showing no observable breakage area.

inversions and other symmetrical rearrangements, that are stable in the sense that they were capable of being transmitted to progeny cells at the time of cell division. Unstable aberrations such as dicentrics, rings, acentric fragments and other asymmetrical rearrangements were observed to a lesser extent Fig. 6.2 shows a metaphase plate, showing chromatid gap Fig. 6.1 reveals a metaphase plate from Group B animals, showing translocation at two sites and centric fusion, at a 3rd site.

According to the classical theory of chromosomal breakage and rejoining, the symmetrical rearrangements should be formed with equal frequencies to asymmetrical rearrangements. This has later been verified using special staining procedures to produce banded chromosomes (Buckton *et al.*, 1978). Structural aberrations (individual + exchange type) were followed by numerical and physiological aberrations. Numerical aberrations are represented by aneuploidy and by polyploidy Fig. 6.3 reveals an aberrant metaphse plate from Group B animals, showing an increased ploidy level. The same photograph also reveals the pulverized nature of some of the chromosomes.

Physiological aberrations include erosion, pulverization and stickyness Fig. 6.4 shows an aberrant metaphase plate from Group B animals (DENA-control), indicating the sticky nature of the chromosomes. In this study DENA produced all the 3 possible varieties of aberrations. Group A animals (normal untreated controls) displayed normal metaphase plates, without any signs of aberration.

Group C animals were administered a single ip injection of DENA and were almost simultaneously treated with chloroform extract of *Trianthema Portulacastrum*. Supplementation of *Trianthema Portulacastrum*, in the diet of Group C animals afforded remarkable protection (Table 6.1) and displayed a remarkably suppressed incidence of DENA induced CA in the cultured leucocytes of rats. The suppressive effect of *Trianthema Portulacastrum* was found to be due to the total length of continuous supplementation, and a maximum beneficial effect was felt after 48 weeks of ip injection of DENA, when karyotypic abnormalities became easily reflected in the blood, Fig. 6.5 reveals a well spread metaphase plate from Group C animal, displaying no observable aberration. *Trianthema Portulacastrum* mediated protection of CA was predominantly reflected in its ability to reduce the structural aberrations, followed by numerical and physiological types.

Abnormal karyotypes from Group B animals and almost normal karyotypes from Group C animals, prompted us to go in for G-banding. The chromosomes were accordingly stained with Giemsa and observed under the microscope for noting differences in the banding patterns of chromosomes in groups B and C. Fig. 6.6 shows G-banded chromosomes of DENA control (Group B) animals, showing numerous breakage areas. Fig. 6.7 shows G-banded chromosomes from Group C animals. No breakage area is seen in the photograph.

In this experiment, the genetic parameters (i.e., aberrations, Karyotyping and G-banding) proved and confirmed once again the Unique anticarcinogenic potential of the $CHCl_3$ extract of *Trianthema Portulacastrum* and also showed for the first time, the remarkable degree of protection afforded by the extract, against the genotoxic effect of DENA a potent hepatocarcinogen. Group D animals (*Trianthema* controls) showed Karyotypic features similar to Group A animals (figure not shown). The long-term experiment showed further, the drastic effects of DENA in inducing C.A's. Out of the 20 animals tested for genotoxicity, all showed aberrant metaphase plates and the incidence of total chromosomal aberrations was 100%. The result was statistically significant. $P<0.001$ compared to Group A animals. By sharp contrast to Group B animals, Group C animals, displayed marked reduction of genotoxicity in terms of reduced rates of CA's -structural, numerical, physiological.

Structural chromosomal aberrations (individual type) dropped to 12% as against 46% in Group B animals and exchange type aberrations were 9% as against 34% in Group B animals. There was a marked reduction in the number of C.A's. Out of the 20 animals tested, not all of them displayed aberrant metaphase plates. Some even showed normal karyotype without any aberration. The total number of C.A's. was just 52 as against 200 in Group B animals and the percentage of C.A. was 26% as against 100% in Group B animals. The extract further could afford a significant degree of protection. The percentage of protection expressed against Group B was 74%.

It has been well established that in majority of the malignant tumours, the neoplastic cells undergo chromosome alterations that are highly complex. A high rate of chromosome breakage (as observed from the G-banded slides) in the experiment are known to be etiologically associated with the initiation of the carcinogenic process. If the breakage lesions are non-random and if the breakage loci happen to be those linked to tumorigenesis, then the probability of tumorigenesis is likely to increase drastically in the target tissue (Dave *et al.*, 1994). In the light of the above, the role of the extract in suppressing the structural and numerical aberrations as observed here, may reflect the ability of the extract to counteract initiations of rat hepatocarcinogenesis. This finding corroborates the earlier observation that the anticarcinogenic potential of *Trianthema Portulacastrum* is maximally observed in the initiation phase of DENA induced rat liver carcinogenesis (Chapter 2).

Regardless of the mechanism of action, it may be concluded that the result of this study provides strong evidence that $CHCl_3$ extract of *Trianthema Portulacastrum* triggers a unique protective effect against induction of C.A's. and karyotypic, anomalies, G-banding patterns etc., under the genotoxic effect of DENA.

The success of these strategies in the animal model systems could eventually be extrapolated to human beings particularly during the early phase of hepatic cancers. This is more specifically relevant, when one considers the ready availability, stability, devoid of toxic side effects, and other positive attributes of the extract, which if given proper therapeutic cognizance, would be able to combat the dreaded killer disease, that has claimed so many lives in the recent past.

References

Arisawa, M., Kinghorn, A.D, Cordell G.A., Farnsworth, N.R. (1983) *J. Nat Prod*, **46**(2), 218-221.

Arisawa, M., Fujita, A., Morita, N., Koshimura, S. (1990) *Planta Medica* **56**, 377-379.

Ashby, J. and Tennant, R.W. (1988) *Mutation Res*, **204**, 17-115.

Aldaz, C.M., Conli, C.J., Klein-Szanto, A.J.P. and Slaga, T.J. (1987) *Proc. Natl. Acad. Sci.* USA, **84**, 2029-2032.

Alberts, D.S. and Garcia, D.J. (1995) *J. Nutr.*, **125**, 692S-697S.

Agarwal, R., Katiyar, S.K., Zaidi, S.I.A. and Mukhtar, H. (1992) *Cancer Res.*, **52**, 3582-3588.

Aquino, T.M., Porta, E.A., Sablan, H.M. and Dorado, R.D. (1985) *Nutr Cancer*, **7**, 25-35.

Ames, B., Holstein, M.C. and Catheart, R. (1982) In : *Lipid peroxides in Biology and Medicine*, Yagi, K. (ed), Academic Press, New York pp. 1-13.

Ames, B. (1983) *Science*, **221**, 1256.

Anderson, E.A. (1985) In : *Methods in enzymology*, Vol. 113, A. Meister (ed), Academic Press, New York, pp. 548-555.

Arias, I.M., Fleischers, G., Kirsch, R., Mischkin, S., Gatmaitan, Z. (1976) In : *Glutathione metabolism and function*, Aris L.M., Jakoby, W.B. (eds), Raven Press, New York, pp. 175-188.

Altman, F.P., Moore, D.S. and Chayen, J. (1975) *J. Histochemistry*, **41**, 227-232.

Arcasoy, M. (1966) *Fed Proc*, **25**, 419.

Biltner, M., Silvia, M., Vargas, J., Bohlmann, A (1983), *Phytochem*, **22**(b), 1523-1524.

Barovada, R., Blasko, G., Shieh, H.L., Pezzuto, J.M. (1990) *Planta Medica*, **56**, 380-382.

Brodt, P. (1996) In : *Cell Adhesion and invasion in cancer metastasis*, Med intelligence, unit, Springer, U.S.A. p. 9.

Bartsch, H., Montesano, R. (1984) *Carcinogenesis*, **5**, 1381-1393.

Bartsch, H., Hictanen, E., Malavelle, C. (1989) *Free Rad Biol Med*, **71**, 637-643.

Biaglow, J.E. (1981) *J. Chem Educ*, **58**, 144-155.

Berenblum, I. and Shubik, P. (1947) *B.J.C.* **1**, 383-386.

Boutwell, R.K. (1964) *Prog. Exp. Tumour Res.* **4**, 207-250.

Bartsch, H., Hictanen, E., Malavelle, C. (1989) *Free Rad Biol Med*, **71**, 637-643.

Blumberg, B.S. (1977) *Science*, U.S.A. **197**, 17-25.

Beer, D.G., Pitot, H.C (1989) *Mutation Res*, **220**, 1-10.

Becker, F.F. (1978) In : *Rat hepatic neoplasia*, Newberne, P.M. and Butler, W.H (eds), MIT Press, Cambridge, M.A, p. 49.

Boone, C.W., Kelloff, G.J. and Malone W.F. (1990) *Cancer Res*, **50**, 2-9.

Bishayee, A., Mandal, A., Chatterjee, M. Chowdhuri, P. (1994) XVI *Int Cancer Congress* 1994, New Delhi, India, Oct. 30th-Nov. 5th, 1994.

Bishayee, A., Chatterjee, M. (1995) *Anticancer Res*, **15**, 455-462.

Bishayee, A., Mandal, A. and Chatterjee, M. (1996) Phytomedicine, **3**, 155-161.

Banerji, A., Chintalawar, G.J., Joshi, N.K. and Chadha, M.S. (1971) *Phytochem*, **10**, 2225.

Bharadwaj, K., Chandra, V. (1987) *Res and Industry*, **32**, 117.

Bannasch, P.L. (1976) *Can Res*, **36**, 2555-2562.

Bannasch, P., Remmer, H., Bolt, H.M. (1978) In : *Primary liver tumours*, Bannasch P. and Popper, H. (eds) MTP Press, Ltd, Lancaster pp. 87-111.

Bhattacharya, S., Chattarjee M. (1998) *Cancer Letters* (In Press).

Bhattacharya, S., Chatterjee, M. (1998) *Italian J. Biochem* (In Press).

Beckman, J.S., Chen, J., Ischiropoulos, H. and Crow, J.P. (1994) In : *Methods in enzymology*, **233**, 229-240.

Bize, I.B., Oberly, L.W., Morris, H.P. (1980) *Can Res*, **40**, 3686-3693.

Bacher, N.R., Gee, M.V., Friedman, R.D. (1982) *Can Res*, **42**, 1078-1081.

Boobis, A.R., Fawthrop, D.J., Davies, D.S. (1987) *Trends Pharmacol Sci*, **10**, 275-280.

Bannai, S. (1984) *Biochim, Biophys Acta,* **779**, 289-300.

Booth, J., Boyland, E. and Sims P. (1961) *Biochem J,* **79**, 516-524.

Boyland, E., Chassaud, L.F. (1969) *Adv Enzmol,* **32**, 172-219.

Benson, A.M., Batzinger, R.P. Ousyl, Bueding E.C., Hay, N., Talalay P. (1976) *Can res,* **38**, 4486-4495.

Benson, A.M., Cha, Y.N., Bueding, E., Heine, H.S., Talalay, P. (1979) *Can Res,* **39**, 2971-2977.

Benson, A.M., Hunkeler, M.J., Morrow, J.F. (1984) *Can Res,* **44**, 5256-5261.

Black, S.D., Coon, M.J. (1989) In : *CytP450, structure, mechanism, biochemistry,* Ortizelle, P.R., Montalleno, D.E. (eds), Plenum Press, New York, pp. 161-216.

Bast, A., Haenan, G.R.M.M. (184) *Trends Biol Sci,* 510-513.

Bock, K.W., Lilienblum, W., Peil, H. and Erickson, L.C. (1982) *Can Res,* **42**, 3747-3752.

Bock, K.W., Kobusch, A.B., Fischer, G.J. (1989) *Can Res Clin oncol,* **115**, 285-289.

Buchmann, A., Kuhhnann, W., Schwartz, M. (1985) *Carcinogenesis,* London, **6**, 513-321.

Benicelli, C., Deflora, S., Camoirano, A. *et al* (1985) *Carcinogenesis,* **6**, 1735-1745.

Basage, M.S. (1989) *Biochem cell Biol,* **68**, 989-998.

Beneditti, A., Casini, A.F., Ferrali, M. and Comporti, M. (1979) *Biochem pharmacol,* **28**, 2909-2918.

Borzio, M., Bruno, S., Mels, G.C., Ramela., G., Borzio, F., Leandro, G., Servida, E. and Podda, M. (1995) *Gastroenterology,* **108**, 812-817.

Buckton, K.E., Hamilton, G.E., Paton, L., Langland, A.O. (178) In : *Mutagen induced chromosome damage in man,* H.J. Evans, D.C. LLoyd (eds) Edinborough Univ, Press, pp. 142-148.

Bodding, P.O. (187) In : *Santhal Medicine* CBN publishers, Calcutta, pp. 09-22.

Ballardini, G., Biolchini, L, Busachi, C.A., and Pisi, E. (1983) *Liver,* **3**, 58-63.

Chen, C., Chan, L., Men, H. (1986) *Hua Hsueh* **44**(2), 61-64.

Constantinides, P. (1984) *Neoplastic response in Ultrastructural pathobiology,* Elsevier, U.S.A. pp. 461-469.

Cooper, D.P., O'Connor, P.J., Bovery, A.C, and Rafferty, J.A. (1995) In : Oxford textbook of oncology, Vol. **1**, Sec 1-7, Peckham, M, Pinedo, M.H. Veroneri, U. (eds), Oxford Univ. Press, U.K.

Curtis, H.J., Tilley, J. (1972) *Radiation Res,* **50**, 539-542.

Columbano, A., Ledda, G.M, Rao, P.M., Rajalakshi, S, and Sarma, D.S.R. (1982) *Cancer Lett*, **16**, 191-196.

Cayama, E., Tsuda, H., Sarma, D.S.R. and Farber, E. (1978) *Nature*, **275**, 60-62.

Chatterjee A., Pakrashi, S. (1994) In : *The Treatise of Indian Medicinal Plants*, Vol. **VI**, Publication and Information Directorate, New Delhi, p. 77.

Chadha, Y.R. (1976) In : The Wealth of India, Raw materials, V-**X**, C.S.I.R, New Delhi, pp. 281-282.

Chopra, R.N., Chopra, I.C., Handa, K.L. (1958) In : *Indegenous drugs of India*, U.N. Dhur and Sons Pvt. Ltd. p. 528.

Cleave, M.J., Hydes, P.C. (1980) Vol. **VII** Siegel H. (ed) pp. 1-62, Marcel Decker, Inc, New York.

Cerrutti, P.A. (1985) *Science*, **227**, 375-381.

Cerrutti, P.A. (1986) In : *Biochem and Mol epiden of cancer*, Harris C.C. (ed), A.R. Liss, New York, pp. 167-176.

Chung, F.L., Hach-Jyun, C.C and Nath, R.G. (1996) *Carcinogenesis*, **17**, 2105-2111.

Cochrane, C.G., Schranfslater, I.U., Hyslop, P., Jackson, J. (1988) In : *O_2 radicals and tissue injury*, Halliwell B (ed) *FASEB* pp. 49-54.

Connor, K.J., Wheeler, L.A. (1987) *Photochemphotobiol* **46**, 239-245.

Cameron, G.R., Karunaratne, W.A.E. (163) *J. Pathol Bacteriol*, **42**, 1-21.

Cameron, G.R., Sweeny, G.D., Jones, K., Lee, G., Farber, E. (1976) *Can Res*, **36**, 3888-3893.

Chasseaud, L.F. (1979) *Adv Can Res* **29**, 175-274.

Christopherson, B.O. (1968) *Biochem J*, **106**, 512-522.

Comporti, M. (1985) *Lab Investig*, **53**, 599.

Cajelli, E., Ferraris, A., Brambilla, G. (1987) *Mutation Res*, **190**, 169-171.

Conney, A.H. (1967) *Pharmacol Rev*, **19**, 317-366.

Cha, Y.N., Haine, H.S. (1982) *Cancer Res* **42**, 2609-2615.

Castuma, C.E., Brenner, R.R. (1989) *Biochem J*, **258**, 723-731.

Crook, L.A., Preiser, F., Cecelia, M. (1991) In : Comprehensive text book of oncology, **VI**, C-32, Moosa, A.R., Stephen, C., Schimpff, F., Robson, M.C. (eds) Williams and Wilkins, Baltimore, p. 254.

Coleman, W., Mc Cullough, K., Esch, G. *et al.*, (1995) *Mol Carcinog*, **13**, 220-232.

Comings, D.E (1975) *Chromosoma*, **50**, 89.

Cole, R.J.N., Taylor, J., Cole, L., Henderson, L. and Arlett, C.F. (1982) *Mutation Res*, **104**, 165-171.

Dragan, Y.P., Hully, J., Nakamura, J., Mass, M.J., Swenberg, J.A. and Pitot, H.C. (1994a) *Carcinogenesis,* **15**, 1451-1458.

Dragan, Y.P., Hully, J., Mass, M.J. and Pitot H.C. (1994b) *Carcinogenesis* **15**, 1939-1947.

Devi, U., P., Ganasoundari, A. (1995) *Ind J. Exp Biol,* **33**, 205-208.

Delucia, A.J., Mustafa, M.G., Hussain, M.Z., Cross, C.U. (1975) *J. Clin Investig,* **55**, 794-802.

Deneke, S.M., Baxter, D.F., Phelps, D.T., Fanburg, B.L. (1989) *Am J. Physiol,* **257**, L265-L271.

Danielson, U.H., Esterbauer, H., Mannervick, K.B. (1987) *Biochem J,* **247**, 707-713.

Dutton, G.S. (1980) In : *Glucuronidation of drugs and other compounds,* C.R.C Press, Boca Raton, Flroida, U.S.A.

Deflora, S. (1978) *Nature* **271**, 455-456.

Deflora, S. (1990) In : *Mechanisms of inhibitors of genotoxicity relevance in preventive medicine,* Mendel Sohn, M.L., Albertini, R.J. (eds), Mutation and Environ, New York, Wiley, Liss, 307-318.

Deflora, S., Aizzotti, A., Agostini, F.D. and Cesarone, C.F. (1991) *Am. J. Med,* **91**, Suppl 3C.

Dillard, D.J., Tappel, A.L. (1979) *Lipids,* **14**, 989-995.

Drochmans, P., Scherer, E. (1972) *J. Cell Biol,* **55**, 63.

Dipaulo, J.A., Popescu, N.C. (1974) *BJC,* **30**, 130.

Drets, M.E., Shaw, M.W. (1971) *Proc Natl Acad Sci,* U.S.A., **60**, 2073.

Dave, B.J., Hsu, T.C., Hong, W.K and Pathak, S. (1994), *Int. J. Oncol,* **5**, 733-740.

Daoust, R. (1963) *Cancer Res Conf,* **5**, 225-239.

El-Deiry, W.S., Tokino, T., Velculescu, V.E., Levy, D.B., Parsons, R., Trent, J.M., Mercer, W.E., Kinzler, K.W. and Vogelstein, B. (1993), *Cell,* **75**, 817.

Epstein, M.A., Holt, S.J. (1963) *J. Cell Biol,* **19**, 325-336.

Epstein, S., Ito, N., Merkow, L., and Farber, E. (1967) *Cancer Res,* **27**, 1702-1711.

Eklowlastbom, L., Rossi, L., Thor, H., Orrenius, S. (1986) *Free Radicals Res Commun* **2**, 57-68.

Ellman, G.L. (1959). *Arch Biochem Biophys* **82**, 70-77.

Esterbaur, H. (1982) In : *Free radicals, lipid peroxidation and cancer,* M.C. Brenner, D.C.H. and Slater, T.F. (eds) Acad Press, London, pp. 101-128.

Esterbaur, H., Zollner, H., Lang, J. (1985) *Biochem J.* **228**, 363-373.

Esterbauer, H., Zollner, H., Schaur, R.J. (1990) In : *Aldehydes formed by lipid peroxidations mechanism of formation, occurrence and determination* Vol. **II** Vigro Pelfrey, C. (ed), membrane lipid oxidation, C.R.C. Press, Boca Raton, Florida, pp. 239-283.

Esterbauer, H., Schaur, R.J. and Zollner, H. (1991) *Free radical Biol Med,* **11**, 81-128.

Eagan, D., James, P., Crook, D., Kennedy, O.R. (1997) *Cancer Lett,* **118**, 201-211.

Emmelot, P., Benedetti, E.L. In : *Some observation on effect of liver carcinogens on the fine structure and function of the E.R of rat cells* in R.J.C. Heim (eds) Protein biosynthesis, Acad Press, New York, pp. 99-133.

Ford, R.J. and Maizel A.L. (1984) In : *Mediators in cell growth and differentiation,* A.L. (eds) Raven Press, New York.

Foulds, L. (1954) *Cancer Res,* **14**, 327-339.

Farber, E. (1973) *Cancer Res,* **7**, 345-375.

Farber, E. (1976a). In : *Liver cell cancer,* Cameron, H.N, Linsell, D.A. and Warwick, G.P. (eds) Elsevier, N. Holland Biomedical Press, Amsterdam. pp. 243-247.

Farber, E. (1976b) *Cancer Res,* **36**, 2532-2533.

Farber, E. Hartman, S. Gruenstein, M. (1976c) *Cancer Res,* **27**, 1702-1711.

Farber, E. (1977) *Cancer Res,* **36**, 2532-2533.

Farber E. (1980a) *Biochim Biophys Acta* **605**, pp. 149-166.

Farber E. Cameron R. (1980b) *Adv Cancer Res,* **31**, 125-126.

Farber, E. (1984a) *Can J. Biochem, Cell Biol,* **62**, 486-494.

Farber, E. (1990) *Biochem Pharmacol,* **39**, 1837-1846.

Fuji, K., Kurata, H., Odashima, S. and Hatsuda, Y. (1976) *Cancer Res,* **36**, 1615-1618.

Firminger, H.I. and Mulay, A.S. (1952) *J. Natl, Cancer, Inst,* **13**, 19-33.

Fiala, S., Fiala, E. and Dixon, B. (1972) *J. Natl. Inst Cancer,* **48**, 1393-1401.

Fiala, S., Fiala, E.S. (1973) *J. Natl Cancer Inst,* **51**, 151-158.

Fazal, U., Razzak, M.A. (1978) In : *Handbook of common remedies in Unani systems of medicine,* C.C.R.U.M, New Delhi, pp 03.

Fridovich, I. (1983) *Ann Rev Pharmacol toxicol,* **23**, 239-257.

Furukawa, T., Meydani S.N. and Blumberg, J.B. (1987) *Mech againg development,* **38**, 107-117.

Fidler, J.J., Hart, I.R. (1982). *Science,* U.S.A. **217**, 998-1003.

Fong, K.L., McCay, P.B., Poyer, J.L. Keele, B.B. and Misra, H.P. (1973) *J. Biol Chem,* **248**, 7792-7796.

Flacks, B., Teh, E.C. (1975) *Chem Biol Interactions* **11**, 277-289.

Ghoshal, S., Singh, S.K. (1986) *J. Chem Res synop* **(3)** 312-313.

Goldfarb, S. (1976) *Cancer Res,* **36**, 2584-2588.

Greenwald, P., Malone, W.F., Cerny, M.E. and Stern, R.H. (1993) In : *Cancer prevention Research trials,* Woude, G.F., Klein, G. (eds) Adv in Cancer Res, Vol. **61**. Acad Press, INC, Harcount Bruce and Co. pp. 1-23.

Garcia, R., Diano, L, Pascale, R. *et al.,* (1989) *Cancer Res,* **49**, 1850-1856.

Gupta, S.K., Bhaskaran, M. (1976) *Ind. J. Pharm,* **38**, 168.

Garg, S.K. (1976) *Ind. J. Med. Res,* **64**, 1133.

Gaettani, G.P., Galiano, S., Canera, L., Ferraris, A.M.,. Kirkman, H.N. (1989) *Blood,* **73**, 334-339.

Gutteridge, J.M.C. (1988) In : O_2 *Radicals and Tissue Injury,* Halliwell, B. (eds) *FACEB* pp. 9-19.

Gutteridge J.M.C., Halliwell, B. (1989) In : *Free radicals in Biol and Med.* Oxford Clarendon Press.

Gutteridge J.M.C. (1993) In *Free Radical Res Commonun* **19**, 141-158.

Glover, J.J. (1990) *J. Natl Cancer Inst,* **82,** 902-903.

Goldstein, B.D., Witz, G, Amoruso, M., Stone, D.S., Troll, W. (1981) *Cancer lett,* 257-262.

Guengerich, F.P. (1990). *Crit Rev Biochem Mol Bio,* **25**, 97-153.

Guengerich, F.P. (1991a) *Chem Res toxicol,* **4**, 391-407.

Gravela, E., Feo, F., Canuto, R.A., Garcea, R., Gabriel, Z. (1975) *Cancer Res,* **35**, 3041-3047.

Glatt, H. (1989) *Mutagenesis,* **4**, 21-227.

Gregus, G., Madhu, C. Klasson, C.D. (1990) *Drug metabolisp,* **18**, 10-19.

Griesemer, A., Squire, A., Stewart, L., Casey, M.W., Murphy D., Nielson, S.W and Stanton, M.F. (1980) *J.N.C.I,* **61**, 183-190.

German, J.L. (1985) In : *Genetics in clinical oncology* Oxford Univ. Press, New York, pp. 3-5.

Gilbert, F. (1983) *J. Natl Cancer Inst,* **71**, 1107-1114.

Grover, S., Fischer, P. (1971) *E.J.C.,* **7**, 77-82.

Gessner, T. (1977) *Cancer Res,* **37**, 2275-2281.

Garfinkel, D. (1958). *Arch Biochem Biophys.* **77**, 493.

Hunt, T. (1991). *Nature,* **350**, 462.

Hatakeyama, M., Herrera, R., Makela, T., Dowdy, S.F., Jack, T. and Weinberg, R.A. (1994). In : *Cancer cell and the cell cycle clock, Mol. Genetics of Cancer,* Vol. **II**, Cold Spring Harbor Lab Press, Cold Spring Harbor symposia on quantitative Biology, U.S.A. pp. 2-9.

Haseltine, W.A. (1983) *Cell,* **33**, 13-17.

Hennings, H., Yuspa, S.H. (1985) *J. Natl Cancer Inst,* **74**, 735-740.

Hennings, H. (1989) In : *Skin carcinogenesis,* Slaga, T.J. Klein-Szanto, A.J.P., Boutwell, R.K., Stevenson, D.E., Spitzer, H.L. and D'Motto, B. (eds) Alan. R. Liss Inc, New York pp. 95-105.

Horsfall, D.J., Tilley, W.D. Orell, S.R. Marshall, V.R. and Cant, E.L.M (1986) *B.J.C.* **53**, 23-28.

Hirota, N., Williams, G.M. (1979) *J. Natl Cancer Inst,* **63**, 1257-1265.

Han, J. (1933) *Prev Med,* **22**, 712-722.

Hertzfeld, A., Greengard, D.C. (1977) *Cancer Res,* **37**, 231-238.

Halliwell, B, Gutteridge, J.M.C. (1989) In : *Free radicals in Biology and medicine,* 2nd Edn Oxford Clarendon Press.

Habig. W.H., Pabst, M.J. and Jakoby W.B. (1974). *J. Biol Chem,* **249**, 7130-7139.

Hayes, J.D., Wolf, C.R. (1988) In : *Glutathione Conjugation,* H-series, Ketterer B. (ed) Acad Press, New York pp. 315-355.

Hammad, H.T., Hagashi N., Tateshi, M., Hanatani and Sakamoto, Y. (1990) *Biochem Biophys acta,* **1055**, 99-106.

Hussain, S.P., Janu, L.N., Rao, A.R. (1990) *Cancer Lett,* **49**, 175-180.

Haenan, G.R.M.M., Bast, A. (1983) *FEBS LETT,* **159**, 24-29.

Hagihara, B., Sato, N., Fukuhara, T., Tsutsumi, K. and Oyangui, Y. (1973) *Cancer Res,* **33**, 2947-2953.

Hirayama, C., Morotomi, I. and Hiroshige, I. (1970) *Biol Chem J,* **118**, 229-232.

Howell, R.R., Stevenson, R.E., Ben-Menachem, Y. Phyliky, R. and Berry, D.H. (1976) *J. Am Med Assoc* **236**, 1481-1484.

Heim, S., Mitelman, F. (1987) *Cancer cytogenetics,* New York, Alan R, Liss 1987.

Horiuchi, T., Kiyoko, I. Minoru, S., Makoto, U. (1984). *Mutation Res,* **140**, 181-185.

Hansen-Melander, E., Melander, Y. and Olin, M.L. (1974) *Hereditas,* **76**, 35.

Hecht, F., Wyandt, H.E. and Mengenis, R.E.H. (1974). In : *The cell nucleus* Vol. 2, Ed H Busch, (ed) Acad Press New York, p. 32.

Itokwa, H., Hirayama, F., Funakoshi, K. and Takeya, K. (1985) *Chem Pharm Bull* **33(8)**, 3488-3492.

Ishikawa, T., Takayama, S., and Kitagawa, T. (1980) *Cancer Res,* **40**, 4261-4264.

Ip, C., El.-Bayoumy, K., Upadhaya, P., Gantha, H., Vandhana Vikit, S., and Thompson, H. (1994) *Carcinogenesis,* **15**, 187-192.

Ip, C. and Lisk D.J. (1994) *Carcinogenesis,* **15**, 1881-1885.

Imlay, J.A., Linn, S. (1988) *Science,* **240**, 640-642.

I.A.R.C. Monographs (1972) Vol. **VI**, Internation Agency for Research on Cancer, Lyon, pp. 107-124.

Ikikawa, T., Marujama, H., Miyano, T., Okura, A., Sawasaki, Y., Oshio, N. *et al.* (1985) *JpN.J. Cancer Res.* **76(2)**, 142-148.

Jorgeo, T., Lu, B., Ocusson, G. (1983) *Tetrahed Lett,* **24(10)**, 1081-1084.

Jing, Y., Ho, G., David, K., Cassady J.M. (1992) *J. Orgchem,* 57, 6198-6202.

Jamwal, S.S.L., Anand, K.K. (1962) *Ind. J. Pharm.* **24**, 218.

Jenkinson, S.G., Spence, T.H., Lawrence, R.A., Hill, K.E., Johnson, K.H. (1987) *J. Apply Physiol,* **62**, 55-60.

Jakoby, W.B., Habig, W.H. (1980) In : *Enzymatic basis of detoxification,* Vol. **12**, W.B. Jakoby (ed) Acad Press, pp. 63-94.

Janu, L.N., Hussain, S.P., Rao, A.R. (1991) *Cancer Lett,* **56**, 59-63.

Kim, R.K., Robbers, J.E., Cheng, K.S. Chung, H.S., Choi, E.C. (1982). *Hanguki, Kyunhakhol Chi,* **10(3)**, 111-117.

Kak, K.B., Chug, H.S., Cheng, K.S., Yang, M.S. (1980) *Hanguki, Kyunhakhol Chi,* **8(2)**, 107-133.

Kaneda, N., Pezzuto, J.M., Kinghorn, A., Douglas, A. (1992) *J. Nat prod* **55(5)**, 654-659.

Kothari, M. and Mehta, L. (1972) In : *Nature of Cancer,* Vol. **VI,** Kothari, Med Pub Co. Bombay, India, pp. 1-8.

Keysser, C.H., Lombard, L.S., Montali, R.J., Stewart, H.L. and Williams, G.M. (1980) In : *Histologic typing of liver tumour of rat.* Nat Acad Sci, Washington D.C. pp. 176-206.

Kirtikar, K.R., Basu, B.D. (1975) In : Indian medicinal plants Vol. **II**, Basu L.M. (ed), Wiley Company Allahabad, India, p. 1180.

Kokpol, U., Nattapol, W.I., Santi, T.P., Warinthorn, C., Gasoon, V., Simpson, J. and Weavers, R. (1997) *Phytochem,* **44**, 719-722.

Kaneko, A., Kimimaro, D., Tohru, K., Shigeaki, Y., Masaki, S., Michio, M. and Tamenorio (1980) *Cancer Res,* **40**, 1658-1662.

Kensler, T.M., Trush, M.A. (1984) *Environ Mutagen* **6**, 593-616.

Kappus, H. (1987) *Chem Phys Lipids* **45**, 105-115.

Ketterer, B., Holt, S.J., Ross Mansell, P. (1967) *Biochem J,* 103, 693-698.

Ketterer, B., Meyer, D.J., Coles, B., Taylor, J.B., Pemble, S. In : *Antimutagensis and anticarcinogenesis mechanisms,* D.M. Shankel, P.E. Hartman, T. Kads, A. Halleander A (eds), Plenum Press, New York, pp. 103-126.

Klingernberg, M. (1958) *Arch Biochem Biophy* **77**, 493.

Kitagawa, A., Sato, H., Sato, K. (1983) *Biochem Biophys Commoun* **112**, 20-28.

Kimbrough, R.D., Linda, R.E., Burse, V.B., Jennings, R.N. (1975) *Arch Environ health,* 392-395.

Karasaki, S.J. (1969) *cell Biol,* **40**, 322-335.

Kitchin, R.M., Louden-Slayer, E.J. (1976) *Stain Tech* **50**, 371.

Kovi, E., and Morris, H.P. (1983) *Adv Enz regul* **14**, 139-162.

Liginsky, W. (1995) *Carcinogenesis,* **16**, 676.

Lapis, K., Beard, D. and Beard, J.W. (1975) *Cancer Res,* **35**, 132-138.

Laishes, B.A., Farber, E. (1978). *J. Natl Cancer Inst,* **61**, 507-512.

Liochev, S.I., Fridovich, I. (1994) *Free Radic Biol Med,* **16**, 29-33.

Loub, W.D., Watanabe, L.W., Davis, D.W. (1975) *J. Natl Cancer Inst,* **54**, 985-988.

Lowry, O.H., Rosenbrough, N.J., Farr, A.L., Randall, R.J. (1985) *J. Biol Chem,* **193**, 265-275.

Lieber, C.S. and De Carli, L.N. (1974) *J. Med Primatol,* **3**, 153-163.

Levine, G. Mierau, G. and Favara, B.E. (1976) *Am. J. Pathol,* **82**, 37.

Luft, J.H. (1961) *J. Biochem Cytol,* **9**, 409-414.

Land, H., Parada, L.F. and Weinberg, R.A. (1983) *Science,* U.S.A. **222**, 771-778.

Levan, A. Levan, G., Mitelaman, F. (1977) *Hereditas,* **86**, 15-30.

Lee, L.W., Tsao, M.S., Grisham, J.W. *et al.* (1989) *Am J. Pathol* **135**, 63-71.

Lee, L.W., Raymond, V.W., Tsao, M.S. (1991) *Cancer Res,* **51**, 5238-5244.

Lee, Y.H., Pank, J.D., Buck, N.L., Kim, S.I., Byung, Z.H. (1995) *Planta Medica* **61**, 178-180.

Lomholt, B., Mohr, J. (1971) *Nature New Biol,* **234**, 109.

Litwack, G., Ketterer, B., Arias, I.M. (1971) *Nature,* **234**, 466-467.

Mudaliar, M., Rao, A. (1958) *Andhra Agric J.* **5**, 153.

Mitscher, L.A., Drake, S., Gollapudi, S.R., Harris, J.A., Shankel, D.M. (1986) In : *Anti mutagenesis and anti carcinogenesis, mechanism,* Shankel D.A., Hartman, P.E., Kada, T., Holleander, A. (eds) Plenum Publishing Corpn, pp. 153-168.

Motokuna, T.T., Bloom, H.J., Kim, H., Juppner, J.V., Ruderman, H.N., Kronenberg, K. and Arnold, A, (1991) *Nature,* **350**, 5-12.

Marx, J.I. (1986) *Science,* U.S.A., **323**, 1093-1095.

Moses, H.L., Yang, D.Y. and, Pietenpol, J.A. (1990) *Cell,* **63**, 245-247.

McCornick, P. Jr., Bertram, J.S. (1982). *Proc Natl Sci,* U.S.A., **79**, 4342-4346.

Miller, J.A., Miller, E.C. (1967) In : *Activation of carcinogenic anomatic amines and amides by N-hydroxylation in vivo in carcinogenesis, a broad criteria,* Williams and Wilkins, Ballimore, pp. 397-420.

Miller, J.A., Miller, E.C. (1976a) *Fed Proc* **35**, 1316-1321.

Miller, E.C. (1978) *Cancer Res,* **38**, 1478-1496.

Miller, S.E., Henderson, B.W. (1986) *Rad Res* **107**, 83-94.

Marquison, G.P., O'Connor, P. (1990) Biol consequences of reactions with DNA : Role of specific lesions in Handbook of Exptal Pharmacology Vol. **94**, Cooper, C.S. and Grover, P.L. (eds) pp. 547-577, Springer Verlage, Berlin.

Marsman, D.S., Popp, J.A. (1994) *Carcinogenesis,* **15**, 111-117.

Mason, T.J., McKay, F.W., Hoover, R., Blot, W.J. and Fraumeni, J.F. Jr. (1976) Atlas of cancer mortality for U.S. countries, 1950-1969 DHEN, Publn No. MIN 75-780, U.S. Deptt of Health, Edn and Welfare, Washington, D.C.

Malone, W.F., Kelloff, G.J., Boone, C.W. and Nixon, D.W. (1989) *Prev Med,* **18**, 553-556.

Mirvish, S.S. (1981a) In : *Inhibition of tumour induction and development,* Zedeck, M.S., and Lipkin, M. (eds) Plenum Publishing Corpn, New York, pp. 101-126.

Mirvish, S.S. (1981b) In : *Cancer Achievements Challenges and Propects for the 1980's,* Burchenal, J.H. and Oeltgen, H.F. (eds) Grune and Stratton New York, pp. 557-558.

Mandal, A., Bishayee, A., Chaterjee, M. (1997) *Phytotherapy Research* (in press).

Mandal, A., Bishayee A., Chaterjee, M. (1997) *Phytomedicine* (in press).

Moreno, F.S., Rizzi, M.B.S.L., Dagli, M.L.Z., Penteado, M.V.C. (1991) *Carcinogenesis* **12**, 1817-1822.

Magee, P.N., Montesano, R., Preussmann, R. (1976) In : *Chem Carcinogens,* Searle C.E. (eds) A.C.S. Monograph series no. 173. Am Chem Soc, Washington, D.C., pp. 491-625.

Micozzi, M.S., Boon, C.W., Kellof, G.L. (1985) *J. Clin Pharmacol,* **25**, 164-175.

Mayskens, F.L. Jr (1988). *J. Natl Cancer Inst,* **80**, 1278-1281.

Moncada, S., Higgs, A.N. (1993) *N. Engl J. Med.* **329**, 2002-2012.

Mochizuchi, Y., Hruben, Z., Morris, H.P., Slesers, A., Vigil, E.L. (1971) *Can Res,* **31**, 763-773.

Marnett, L.J., Tuttle, M.A. (1980) *Cancer Res,* **40**, 276-282.

Meister, A. (1982) In : *Current topics in cellular regulation* Vol. **X** Acad Press, New York, pp. 21-58.

Meister, A., Anderson, M. (1983) *Ann Rev Biochem* **52**, 711-760.

Mannervick, V. (1985) *Adv enzymol relat aneas, Mol Biol,* 357-417.

Manson, M.M., Ketterer, B. (1988) In : *Carcinogenic and mutagenic responses to aromatic amines and nitroarenes,* Elsevier, R. Press, Amsterdam, pp. 303-314.

Moorghen, M., Cairns, J., Forrester, L.M., Hayes, A.K., Lattan, A.R., Wolf, C.R., Harris, A.L. (1991) *Carcinogeneis* **12**, 13-17.

Mudler, G.J. (1992) *Ann Rev Pharmacol Toxicol,* **32**, 25-49.

Meyer, D.J., Beale, D., Hong, T., K.H., Coles, B. and Ketterer, B. (1985). *FEBS Lett,* **184**, 139-143.

Merill, J.C., Bray, T.N. (1982) *Can. J. Physiol, Pharmacol,* **60**, 1556-1561.

Morse, M.A., Stoner, G.D. (1995) *Carcinogenesis,* **16**, 973.

Mukherjee, K.L. (1988) In : Medical lab Tech - A procedure manual for routine diagnostic tests Vol. **III** Tata McGraw Hill, New Delhi, pp. 1126-1171.

Miyaji, T. (1976) *Gann. Monogr. Cancer Res,* **18**, 129-149.

Mistry, K.J., Krishna, M., Bhatacharya, R.K. (1997) *Cancer Lett,* **121**, 99-104.

Masahiro, T., Kazuo, O., Toshifumi, T. *et al.* (1996) *JpN. J. Cancer Res,* **87**, 5-9.

Matsuoka, A., Hayashi, M., and Ishidate, M. Jr. (1979) *Mutation Res,* **66**, 277-290.

Mitelman, F., Hein, S. (1990) *Cancer Prev.* **14**, 527-540.

Matsui, S.I., Sasaki, M.S. (1975) *Japan J. of genetics,* **50**, 189.

Nowell, N.P. (1976) *Science,* **194**, 23-28.

Nowell, P.C. (1986) *Cancer Res,* **46**, 2203-2207.

Noble, R.L. (1977) *Cancer Res,* **37**, 82-94.

Newberne, P.M., Wogan, G.N. (1968) *Cancer Res,* **28**, 770-780.

Newmark, H., Mergens, W. (1981) In : *Inhibition of tumour induction and development* Zedec, M.S. and Lipkin, M. (eds) Plenum Publishing Corpn, New York, pp. 127-168.

Nayar, R.C. (1980) Second Scientific Seminar of C.C.R.U.M. Bombay.

Nakayama, T., Kimura, T., Kodama, N., Nageta, C. (1983) *Carcinogenesis,* **4**, 765-769.

Nijhoff, W.A., Green, G.N., Peters, W.H.N. (1993) *International J. Mol.* **3**, 1131-1139.

Novi, A.M. (1981) *Science,* **212**, 541.

Newmann, C.M., Zanoi, V.G. (1990a) *Biochem J.* **258**, 723-731.

Newmann, C.M., Zanoi, V.G. (1990b) *Biochem Pharmacol,* **39**, 1085-1093.

NourEl-deen, A.F., Craig, M.M. and Gresser M.J. (1985) *J. Biol Chem,* **260**, 6836-6842.

Natarajan, A.T., Tates, A.D., Van Burl, P.P.W. *et al.* (1976) *Mutation Res* **37**, 83-90.

Ogawa, K., Solt, D.B., and Farber, E. (1980) *Cancer Res*, **40**, 725-733.

Oberly, L.W., Oberly, T.D. (1986) In : *Free radicals ageing and degenerative diseases*, Johnson, J.E., Waford. R., Harman, D., Mitchel, J. (eds) A.R. Liss, New York, pp. 325-371.

Omura, T., Sato, R. (1964) *J. Biol Chem*, **239**, 2370-2377.

Okhawa, H., Ohishi, N. and Yagi, K. (1979) *Anal Biochem*, **95**, 351-358.

Oyangui, Y., Sato, N. and Hagihara, B. (1974) *Cancer Res*, **34**, 456-462.

Otmar, S., Clauss, S., Grudman, W. (1981) *Phytochem* **20(8)**, 1983-1985.

Porten, J. (1974) In : *Carcinogenesis in vitro*, Grundmann, E. (ed) Springer Verlag, Berlin, pp. 43-47.

Pitot, H.C., Barness, L., Goldsworthy, T., Kitagawa, T. (1978a) *Nature*, **271**, 456-458.

Pitot, H.C. (1978b) In : *The induction of drug metabolism* Esterbauer, K.R.W. and Lidenbarb, E. (eds) Schalt Verlag, Struggart, pp. 471-483.

Pitot, H.C., Sirica, A.E. (1980) *Biochim Biophy Acta*, **605**, 191-215.

Pitot, H.C. (1986a) In : *Fundmantals of Oncology Marcel* Dekker, Inc, New York.

Pitot, H.C. (1987) Sym Fund *Cancer Res*, **39**, 187-196.

Pitot, H.C., Campbell, H.A. and Maronpot, R. (1989) *Toxicol, Pathol*, **17**, 594-605.

Pitot, H.C., Dragan, Y.P. (1991) *FACEB J.*, **5**, 2280-2286.

Periano, C., Fry, R.J.M. and Staffeldt, E. (1971) *Cancer Res*, **31**, 1506-1512.

Peiano, C., Fry, R.J.M. and Grube, D.D. (1978) In : *Carcinogenesis mechanisms of tumour promotiion and carcinogenesis*, Slass, T.J., Slivaw and Boutwell, R.W., (eds) Raven Press, New York, pp. 421-432.

Periano, C., Richards, W.L. and Stevens, F.J. (1989) In : *Mechanisms of tumour promotion* Vol. **1**, T.J Slaga (eds) pp. 1-53, CRC Press, Boca Raton, Florida.

Prince, M., Hitachi, K., Yamada, Takayama, S. (1974) *J. Natl Can Inst*, **53**, 507-516.

Preusessmann R. (1975) In : Handbook of pathol, B.D., V 1/2 Teilz, Springer, Verlag, Berlin, Hidelberg and New York.

Preusessmann, R. (1978) In : *Primany liver tumour* Remeer, H., Bolrhv Bannasch, P. and Popper, H. (eds) MTP Press L.T.D. Lancaster pp 11-29.

Popper, H., Maltoni, C., Selikof, I.J., Squire R.A., Thomas, L.B., (1977) In : Cold Spring Harbor Conferences on Cell Proliferation, Vol. **4**, *Origin of human cancer*, Cold Spring Harbor Press, New York, p. 1359.

Popper, H. (1978) In : *Primary liver tumors* Remmer, H., Boll. Bannash, P., Popper, H. (eds); M.T.P., Press Ltd. Lancaster p. 8.

Perchellet, J.P., Owen, M.P., Posey, T.D., Orten, D.K., Schneider. V.A. (1985) *Carcinogenesis,* **6**, 567-573.

Perchellet, J.P., Percehllet, E.M. (1989) *Free Radical Biol Med,* **7**, 377-408.

Pascale, R.M., Simile, M.M., Satta, G. *et al.* (1991) *Anticancer Res,* **113**, 1617-1624.

Parikh, D., Daniel, M. (1990) *Ind. J. Pharm Sci,* **54**, 73.

Peskin, A.V., Koen, Y.M., Zbansky, I.B. (1977) *FEBS Lett,* **78**, 41-45.

Palozza, P., Agostini, G., Picconi E., Bardoli, G. (1994) *Arch Biochem Biophys* **312**, 88-94.

Parker, C.W., Fishman, C.M., Wedner, H.J. (1980) *Proc Natl, Acad Sci,* U.S.A. **77**, 6870-6873.

Pearson, W.R., Windle, J.J., Morrow, J.F., Benson, A.M., Talalay, P. (1983) *J. Biolchem,* **258**, 2052-2062.

Porter, K.R., Bruni, C.C. (1959) *Cancer Res,* **19**, 997-1009. Peste Alexander Reeve.

Porter. T.D., Coon, M.J. (1991) *J. Biol Chem,* **266**, 13469-13472.

Paolini, M., Legator, M.L. (1992) *Nature,* **357**, 448.

Pickett, C.B., Tlakowski, Hopkins, C.A. Ding, G.I.F. *et al.* (1984) *J. Biol Chem,* **259**, 5182-5188.

Pickett, C.B., Tlakowski, Hopkins, C.A., Ding, G.I.A., Ding, V.D.H. and King, B.G. (1987) In : *GST and Carcinogenesis.,* Martle, T.T., Pickett C.B., Hayes, T.D. (eds) Taylor and Francis, London, pp. 75-85.

Pantuck, E.J., Hsio, K.C., Loub, W.D., Watternberg, L.W., Kalzymer, R., Conney, A.H. (1976) *J. Pharmacol Exp, Thera* **277**, 283.

Poli, G., Albano, E. and Dianzani, M.U. (1987) *Chem Phys Lipids,* **45**, 117-120.

Pryor, W.A. (1978) *Photochem Photo Biol,* **28**, 787-801.

Paolini, M., Mesirca, R., Delucia, C., Baur, C., Biagi, G.L., Canetelli-Forti, G. (1995) *Carcinogenecis,* **16**, 971-972.

Pearse, A.G.E. (1985) In : Histochemistry theoretical and applied Vol. **II**, Analyst Tech, Churchill livingstone, U.K. pp. 538-540.

Puchtler, H., Sweat, F., Kuhns, J.G. (1964) *J. Histochem, Cyto Chem,* **12**, 900.

Priest, J.H. (1969) In : *Med Tech Series, Cytogenetics Lea and Febinger,* P.A. pp. 53-67.

Ren, D.L., Wang, J.Z., Noda, H., Amano, H., Ogawa, S. (1995) *Planata Medica,* **61**, 120-125.

Rous, P. and Kidd, J.C. (1941) *J. Expt, Med,* **73**, 365-376.

Rotello, R.J., Liebermann, R.C., Purchio, A.F. and Gerschenson, L.E. (1991) *Proc Natl Acad Sci,* U.S.A., **88**, 3412-3415.

Reuber, M.D. (1965) *J. Natl Cancer Inst,* **34**, 697-723.

Rao, P.N., Lawrier, C., Nagamine, Y., Roomi, M.W., Rajalakshi, S. and Sarma, D.S.R. (1983) *Proc Am Asso Cancer Res,* **24**, 86.

Rana, M.P., Sardar, S. and Chatterjee, M. (1998a) *Mol Cell Biochem* (In Press).

Rana, M.P., Sardar, S., Chaterjee, M. (1998b) Tumour Biol. (In Press).

Ravishankar, V., Mehta, A.K. (1979) *J. Nat prod,* **42**, 152.

Rabes, H.L., Scholze, P., Jantsch, B. (172) *Cancer Res,* **32**, 2577-2586.

Roltstein, J.B., Slaga. T.J. (1988) **202**, 421-427.

Reiners, J.J. Jr., Kodasi, E., Cappel, R.E. and Gilbert, H.F. (1991) *Carcinogenesis,* **12**, 2345-2352.

Reynolds, E.S. (1963) *J. Cell Biol,* **17**, 208.

Rowley, J.D., Golomb, H., Vardiman, J., Fukuhara. S. *et al.* (1977) *I.J.C,* **20**, 869-872.

Rowley, J. (1980) *Can Genet Cytogen* **2**, 175-198.

Stoker, M. (1996) In : *Fundamantals of Cancer Cell Biol,* Adv Can Res, Vandwondegt, Klein G. (eds) Acad Press, SanDiego, U.S.A. pp. 11-12.

Shelby, M.D. and Stasiewicz, S. (1984) *Environ mutagen,* **6**, 871-878.

Sargent, L., Xu, Y.H., Sattler, G.L., Meisner, L. and Pitot, H.C. (1989) *Carcinogenesis,* **10**, 387-391.

Sargent, L.M., Sattler, G.L., Roloff. B. *et al.* (1992) *Cancer Res,* **52**, 955-963.

Sasaki, T., Yoshida, T. (1935) : *Virch Arch Pathol Anat Physiol* **295**, 175-200.

Stenback, W.A., Anderson, J.P., McCormick, K. and Trentin, J.J. (1973) *J. Natl Cancer Inst,* **50**, 963-970.

Sherlock, S. (1974) In : *Toxic liver injury,* Farber, E. and Fishcer, M.M. (eds) Marcel Dekker, Inc, New York.

Sherlock, S. (1979) *Cancer Res,* **36**, 2584-2588.

Squire, R.A., Levitt, M.H. (1975) *Cancer Res,* **35**, 3214-3223.

Sell, M.A., Katyal, S.L., Sell, S., Shinozuka, H. and Lombardi, B. (1979) *B.J.C.* **40**, 274-283.

Sell, S. (1990) *Cancer Res,* **50**, 3811-3815.

Solt, D., Farber, E. (1976) *Nature,* **263**, 701-703.

Solt, D.B., Medline, A. and Farber, E. (1977) *Am J, Pathol,* **88**, 595-618.

Shinozuka, H., Sells, M.A., Katyal, S.L., Sell, S., Lombardi, B. (1979) *Cancer Res,* **39**, 2515-2521.

Scherer, E., Stewart, A.P., Emmelot, P. and Friedrich, F. (1972) *J. Natl Cancer Inst*, **49**, 93-106.

Scherer, E., Emmelot, P. (1975a) *E.J.C.*, **11**, 145-157.

Scherer, E., Emmelot, P. (1975b) *E.J.C.*, **11**, 689-696.

Scherer, E., Emmelot, P. (1976) *Can Res*, **36**, 2544-2554.

Scherer, E., Hoffmann, M. (1977) *E.J.C.*, **7**, 369-371.

Scherer, E. (1984). *Biochim Biophys Acta*, **738**, 219-236.

Sirica, A.E., Barness, L., Goldsworthy, T. and Pitot, H.C. (1978) *J. Environpathol toxicol*, **2**, 21-28.

Slaga, T.J., Solanki, W. and Loghni, N. (1983) In : *Radioprotectors and Anticarcinogens* Nygaards, O.F. and Simig, M.G. (eds) Academic Press, I.N.C. New York, pp. 417-485.

Sen, K.C., Ray, S.N., Ranjhan, S.K. (1978) I.C.A.R. publications, N. Delhi.

Singh, B.P., Jha O.P., Ghosh, P.K. (1982a) *Plant Physiol Biochem*, **9**, 14.

Singh, B.P., Singh, R.P., Jha, O.P. (1982b) *Biol Bulletin of India*, **4**, 157.

Stewart, H.L., Williams, G.H., Keyesser, C.H., Lombardi, L.S., Montali, R.J. (1980) *J. Natl. Can Inst* **64**, 177-207.

Sarkar, A., Mukherjee, B., Chatterjee, M. (1994a) *Carcinogenesis*, **15**, 1055-1060.

Swenberg, J.A., Hoel, D.G. and Magee, P.N. (1991) *Can Res*, **36**, 6409-6414.

Sato, K., Kitagawa, A., Sato, H. *et al.* (1984) *Gann*, **75**, 199-202.

Sato, T., Takasagawa, K., Soo, N., Konno, K., Thuku J. (1989) *J. Exp. Med*, 138, 445-461.

Sato, K. (1990) *Adv Can Res*, **52**, 205-255.

Slaga, T.J., Szrnto, A.J.P., Triplett, L.C. and Yotti, L.P. (1981) *Science*, **213**, 1021-1022.

Smith, T.M., Thor, H., Hantzol, P. and Orrenius, S. (1982) *Biochem Pharmacol*, **31**, 19-26.

Slater, T.F., Sawyer, B.C. (1971) *Biochem J.*, **123**, 805-814.

Streeter, A.J., Dahlin, D.C., Nelson, S.D., Baillie T.A. (1984) *Chem Biol interaction*, **48**, 349-366.

Shaw, J.P., Chow, I.N. (1986) In : *J. Cell Physiol*, **129**, 193-198.

Sparnins, V.L., Venegas, P.L., Wattenberg, L.W. (1982) *J. Natl Cancer Inst*, **68**, 493-496.

Salmon, J.A., Cohen, E., Cohen, C., Bengbson, G. (1974) *Histochemistry*, 42, 61-74.

Stark, A.A., Zeger, E., Pagano, D.A. (1988) *Carcinogenesis*, **9**, 771-777.

Slater, T.F. (1984) *Biochem J.* **222**, 1-5.

Swinger, B.A., Buge, J.A., O' Neal, F.O. and Aust, S.D. (1979) *J. Biol Chem,* **254**, 5892-5899.

Schabadasch, A.L. (1947) *Proc Nat Acad Sci,* U.S.S.R. Ser, Biol, **6**, 745.

Spycher, M.A., Gitzelman, R. (1971) *Virch Arch, B,* **8**, 133-139.

Svoboda, D.J. (1964) *J. Natl Cancer Inst,* **33**, 315-340.

Svoboda, D.J. and Higginson, J. (1968) *Can Res,* **28**, 1703-1733.

Sabatini, D.C., Bennasch, K. and Barnett, R.J. (1963) *J. Cell Biol,* **17**, 19-58.

Smuckler, E.A., Arcasoy, M. (1969) *Int Rev Exp pathol,* **7**, 305-418.

Solomon, E., Borrow, J. and Goddard, A.D. (1991) *Science,* **254**, 1153-1161.

Sharma, A.K., Sharma, A. (1980) Chromosome Techniques, Theory and Practice, Butterworth London, pp. 409-425.

Schendel, W. (1973) *Nobel Symposium,* **23**, 342.

Seabright, M. (1972) *Chromosoma* **36**, 204.

Summer, A.T., Evans, H.J. and Buckland, R.A. (1973) *Exptal Cell Res,* **81**, 214.

Sarkar, A., Mukherjee, B., Rana, M.P., Chatterjee, M. (1994b) *Cancer Investing,* **12**, 477-483.

Takemoto, T., Nishimoto, N., Nakai, S., Takagi, N., Hayashi, S., Odashima, S., Wada, Y. (183) *Tett Lett,* **24(10)**, 1057-1060.

Tantivatana, P., Ruangrungri, N., Vaisinirag V. *et al.* (1983) *J. Orgchem* **48(2)**, 268-270.

Tantishaiyakal, V., Pumangura, S., Chaichan, T.C., Mawen, W., Mc. Laughten, J.L. (1986) *J. Nat Prod,* **49(1)**, 180-181.

Takeuchi, S., Konoyoshi, K., Hadiman, N. *et al.* (1986) *Biochem,* **50(3)**, 569-573.

Tsuda, H., Farber, E. (1979) *Proc Am Assoc Cancer Res,* **20**, 61.

Tsuda, H., Uehara, N., Iwahari, Y. *et al.* (1994) *JpN.J. Can Res,* **85**, 1214-1219.

Tatematsu, M., Murasaki, G., Nakanishi, K., Miyata, Y., Shinozuka, Y. and It, N. (1979) *JpN J. Can. Res.* **70**, 125-130.

Turosov, V.S., Deningev, M.W., Dunn, T.B., Stewart, H.L. (1973) *J. Nat Can Inst,* **51**, 1689-1696.

Thompson, H.J., Meeker, L.D., Kokosha, S. (1984) *Cancer Res,* **44**, 2083-2086.

Tso, P.O., Caspany, W.J., Lorentzen, R.J. (1977) In : *Free radicals in biology* Vol. **3**, Pryor. (eds) Acad Press, New York, pp. 251-303.

Troll, W., Weisner, R. (1985) *Ann Rev Pharmacol Toxicol,* **25**, 509-528.

Tan, K.H., Mayer, D.J., Coles, B., Ketterer, B. (1986) *FEBS Letts,* **207**, 231-233.

Totter, J.B. (1980) *Proc Natt Acad Sci,* U.S.A. **77**, 1763-1967.

Talalay, P., Batzinger, R.P., Benson, A.M., Bueding, E., Cha, Y.N. (1979) *Adv Enz regul,* **17**, 23-26.

Tephly, T.R., Burchell, B. (1990) *Trends Pharmacol Sci,* **11**, 276-279.

Teebor, G.N., Becker, F.F. (1971) *Cancer Res,* **31**, 1-3.

Toshifumi, T., Masahiro T., Akira, K. *et al.* (1996) *Jpn J. Can Res,* **87**, 111-115.

Testa, R.T. (1991) In : *Comprehensive textbook of oncology,* A.R. Moosa, Schimpff, M.C., Robson (eds) Williams and Wilkins, pp. 81-83.

Tsao, M.S., Smith, J., Nelson, K., Grisham, J.A. (1984) *Exptal Cell Res,* **154**, 38-52.

Tsao, M.S., Grisham, J., Nelson, K. and Smith, J. (1985) *Am J. Pathol,* **118**, 306-315.

Trusler, S. (1975) *Lancet,* **I,** 44.

Tates, A.D., Neuteboone, I., Hoffker, M. and Den Englese, L. (1980) *Mutation Res,* **74**, 11-20.

Ulubelen, A., Oksuz, S. (1982) *J. Nat Prod,* **45(3),** 373.

Uhlig, S., Wendel, A. (1982) *Life Science,* **51**, 1083-1094.

Vang, O., Rasmussen, F., Anderson, O. (1997) *Cancer Lett,* **114**, 283-286.

Vahakangas, K., Haigen, A., Nasris, C.C. (1985) *Carcinogenesis* **6**, 1169-1176.

Vohra, S.B., Shah, S.A., Naqvi, S.A.H., Ahmed, S., Khan, M.S.Y. (1983) *Planta medica,* **47**, 106-108.

Vass, L., Sellyee, M. (1972) *Lancet* **II,** 1093.

Vass, L., Selleye, M. (1973) *Humangenetik* **18**, 81.

Valisolalao, J., Lu, B., Occusson, G. (1983) *Tetrahed Lett,* **39(17)**, 2779-2785.

Van Duren, B.L., Sivak, A, Katz, C., Seidman, I., Melchionne, S. (1975) *Can Res,* **35**, 502-505.

Wall, M.E., Krieder, M.M., Kruwson, C.F., Eddy, C.R., Willman, J.J., Correll, D.S. and Gentry, H.S. (1954a). *J. Am Pharm Assoc,* Scieds **43**, 1-7.

Wall, M.E., Eddy, C.R., Willman, J.J., Correl, D.S., Schubert, B.G., and Yentry, H.S. (1954b). *J. Am Pharm Assoc (Scied)* **43**, 503-505.

Wall, M.E., Rendke, C.S., Kenney, H.E., Willaman, H.E., Correll, J.J *et al.* (1957) *Am Pharm Assoc (Scied)* **46**, 653-684.

Wall, M.E., Garwin, J.W. Willaman, J.J., Jones, G. *et al.* (1961) *J. Pharm Sci,* **50**, 1001-1034.

Wall, M.E., Wani, M.C. (1967) In : *Recent progress in plant anti tumour agents,* 153rd National Meeting of Ancham.

Wall, M.E., Wani, M.C., Natscake, S.M., Nicholas, A.W. (1986) *J. Med Chem,* **29(8)**, 1953-1955.

Wall, M.E., Wani, M.C. (1995) *Can Res,* **55**, 753-760.

Woodbury, A.M., Wall, M.E., Willasman, J.J. (1961) *J. Econ Bot,* **15**, 79-86.

Wenger, B., Italiano, L., Beck, J.P., Bastidia, J., Bergonon, S., Codina, C., Lobstein. A., Anton, R. (1995) *Planta Medica,* **61**, 77-79.

Wickramaratne, B.N., Mar, W., Choi, H., Castillo, J.J., Farnsworth, W.R., Soejarto, D.D., Cordell, G.A., Pezzuto, J.M., Kinghorn A.D. (1995) *Planta Medica,* **61**, 80-81.

Wani, M.C., Taylor, H.I., Wall, M.E. *et al.* (1971) *J. Anchem Soc,* **93**, 2325-2327.

Weinberg, R.A. (1985) *Science,* U.S.A., **230**, 770-776.

Wattenberg, L.W. (1972) *Toxicol appl pharmacol,* **23**, 741-748.

Wattenberg, L.W. (1975) *J. Natl Can Inst,* **54**, 1005-1006.

Wattenberg, L.W., Hanley, A.B., Baranj, G., Sparnings, V.L., Lam, L.W.T., Fenwick, G.R. In : Diet Nutrition and Cancer.

Watternberg, L.W. (1978) *J. Natl Can Inst,* **54**, 1005-1006.

Wattenberg, L.W., Lam, L.K.T. (1984) In : Banbury report, 17, Coffee and Health, Cold Spring Harbor Press, New York, pp. 137-145.

Watternberg, L.W (1985) *Can Res,* **45**, 1-3.

Wattenbeg, L.W. (1985) *Can Res,* **45**, 1-8.

Wattenberg, L.W. (1992) *Can Res,* **52**, 2085-2091.

Wattenberg, L.W., Hanley, A.B., Baranj, G, *et al.* In : *Diet Nutrition and Cancer Hayashi,* Y. Mago, N. (eds) Jpn Sc, Soc, Tokyo, V and U Press pp. 193-203.

Williams, G.M., Yamomoto, R.S. (1972) *J. Natl, Can, Inst.* **49**, 685-692.

Williams, G.M., Kloiber, M., Pankev, S.E. and Farber, E. (1976) *J. Natl Can Inst,* **57**, 157-165.

Williams, G.M., Watanabe, K. (1978) *J. Natl, Can Inst,* **61**, 113-118.

Williams, G.M., (1980a) *Biochem Biophys Acta,* **605**, 167-189.

Williams, G.M., (1980b) *Biochem Biophys Acta,* **605**, 191-215.

Wood, A.W., Haong, M.T., Chang, R.L. *et al.* (1982) *Proc Natl Acad Sci,* U.S.A., **79**, 5513-5517.

Wahid, A., Siddiqui, H.H. (1961) In : *A survey of drugs institute of history of medicine and medical research,* pp. 110-135, pp. 150-158.

Waitzberg, D.L., Gonsalvez, E.L., Fintuch, J., Bevillacoua, I.R., Roca, C.L., Dogni (1989) *Brazil J. Med. Biol Res,* **22**, 447-455.

Wuh, Y., Lin, J.K. (1995) *Anal Chem,* **67**, 1603-1612.

Wood, J.L. (1970) In : *Metabolic conjugation and metabolic hydrolysis* Vol. **II** Fisherman, W.H. (ed) Acad, Press, New York, pp. 261-299.

Woodruf, M.F.A. (1983) *B.J.C.* **47**, 589-594.

Wislocki, P.G., Mowa, G.T. Lu, A.Y.N. (1980) In : *Enzymatic basis of detox fication* Vol. **I**, Jakoby, W.B. (eds), Acad press, New York, pp. 135-182.

Watanabe, K., Williams, G.M. (1978) *J. Natl Can Inst*, **61**, 1311-1314.

Wada, S., Kato, T., Mutai, K., Kozaki, K., Yamaguchi, S., Kim, J., Toriyama, B.H., Asamoto, M., Ita, N., Tsuda, H. (1996) *Jpn J. Can Res*, **87**, 240-246.

Wolman, S., Harland, A. and Becter, F. (1972). *J. Natl Cancer Inst*, **46**, 1261-1269.

Yoshiyoka, Y., Tabeta, R., Sato, H., Hazine, B., Vehara, N., Fukuka, F. (1985) *Carbohydrate Res*, **140(1)**, 93-100.

Yuspa, S.H., Harris, G.C. (1982) In : Cancer epidemiology and prevention, Schotten D. and Fraumani, J.F. (eds). W.B. Saundr Co. Philadelphia, pp. 23-43.

Yuspa, S.H., Poirier, M.C. (1988) *Adv. Cancer Res*, **50**, 25-70.

Yuspa, S.H. Hennings, H., Roop, D., Strickland, J. and Green Halgh, D.A. (1990) In. *Genetic mechanisms in carcinogeneis and Tumou progression*, Harris, C.C., Liotta (eds), Wiley Lis, New York, pp. 115-126.

Yoshiji, H., Nakae, D., Kinugasa, T., Matsuzati, M., Denda, A., Tsuzi, T., Konixhi, Y. (1991) *B.J.C.*, **64**, 839-842.

Yin, H., Benetti, G., Jones, J.P. (1994) *Chem Biol Interactions*, **90**, 47-58.

Yagi, K. (1991) In : New Trends in Biochem, Ozawa, T. (eds), Spriner, Verlag, Berlin, pp. 207-223.

Yunis, J.J., Sanchez, O. (1975) *Humangenetik*, **27**, 167.

Zuckerman, A.J. (1978) In : *Primary liver tumours*, Remmer, T., Bolt, H.M., Bannasch, P. and Popper, H. (eds) MTP Press Ltd. Lancaster, pp. 425-429.

Zakim, D., Cantor, M., Etil, H. (1988) *J. Biol Chem*, **263**, 5164-5169.

Zimmermann, J.J, Gorski, J.P., Kasper, C.B. (1977) *Drug Metab, Diagnos*, **5**, 572-578.

INDEX